My Journey - Conceiving Pregnancy Delivery

The journey that shows you

what love is!

By

Jaimala Wankhede Shetty

ISBN: 979886977084

PREFACE

I am no doctor nor a birthing counsellor but I am a first-time mom who researched before and through the pregnancy journey. There are quite a lot of things that I experienced during my pregnancy and there are some that I read about but did not personally experience. I am also part of a lot of mommy and mommy-to-be groups which helped me learn from the experiences of others. When I started this journey, I did not know how it would be, whether I would be able to handle it but the researcher in me kept researching to always be prepared mentally and physically for this new me. As I progressed in my journey and gained more knowledge, I always felt the need to share it with other would-be moms. I know there are a lot of books on these topics in the market but still I wanted to do my bit by sharing my knowledge. Also, most of the resources that I came across were lengthy so I thought of writing this book by keeping the information delivery crisp.

The plan for this book is to share my real-life experience of conceiving, pregnancy and then having the baby. But also, to share knowledge around some of the Indian home-remedies/easy solutions that helped me and others to take care of some pregnancy issues. While the book has general pregnancy related information, there are some recommendations or mentions that might be Indian related.

ACKNOWLEDGMENTS

I cannot imagine being able to survive the pregnancy and the post-delivery period with the baby and my health without my husband. He has been my biggest strength throughout. Second on the list of thank you is my son. A lot of this book has been written while breastfeeding him in the nights, thanks to him who gave me all these experiences and so I could incorporate those in this book.

My mom, my mother-in-law, my father-in-law and sister-in-law who enquired about me each day and kept a tap on me and my health all through the pregnancy and posted it. With these people around, I knew I am loved and cared for ♥ □.

My book reviewers - Prashant Shetty, Sneha Shetty and Vedika Sonawane, thank you for your valuable feedback and helping shape the book better.

1. Decision of Giving it a Try

The day you decide you are going to have a baby, from that day your life changes. It is such a big decision that you can never be fully-prepared to take the leap. It is a life changing experience that no matter how much ever you think about it, you never surely know the answer. Being a millennial, the decision wasn't easy for me and my partner either. We had lived our life on our own terms all this while, working like crazy, vacationing when we wanted - no barriers to what we could do. And now we were here, where we wanted to decide whether we wanted to bring this tiny-being into the world, and make it grow in the best possible way!

Being above 30 and having always heard, oh you can't conceive easily post 30, we also wondered if we really wanted to take that stress?

Finally, after much debate, we decided we wanted to give it a try. The first time we had unprotected sex, I freaked out at the thought of this big responsibility and we again decided to wait for a little more. After giving ourselves some time, about 3 months later from the first try - we decided we wanted to give this a go. And then starts the journey of endless nervous/anxiety sex, crazy pregnancy tests and wondering endlessly on what and how to do it right so that you conceive.

Now once we decided we wanted to give it a try, we went to our family doctor just to see if we should do any tests (vitamin, mineral deficiency kinds) before we start. The doctor said we were in a healthy age [up to the age of 35 years, a female is considered most fertile] with no diseases so we should just begin to try and I should start taking folic acid tablets as it gives energy needed for this journey. The folic acid tablet started now while trying to conceive should be taken for the whole of the first trimester and some doctors even ask women to continue it until the second trimester.

When we started trying, the initial first month was super fun. Having regular sex, trying to enjoy it and then waiting nervously to take the test. My body hormones started playing up quite a bit from the first month of non-protective sex.

My periods are usually regular but this month they were delayed by like 10 days - oh man, it got me all hopeful. And why not, it takes only one sperm to swim through to make it happen. After about 9 days of delay in the period, I took the test and huh it came out negative. I was disappointed but hopeful, maybe I tried it too early. My hopefulness did not have to stay long, the next day I got my periods, as though it was waiting for me to test.

With the first month of my failed attempt, the researcher in me started exploring what can be done, how to best conceive, I posted queries on a couple of my Facebook & WhatsApp Mammas groups. There was a lot of advice I got on my queries but one advice that an Asian lady gave which is immensely valuable (I realized it only later). She said enjoy having sex, don't go for sex thinking it is to have the baby. Try to do fun things, pole dance, role-play or whatever you guys fancy and make it fun. But when you are at the start of this baby journey, it is really difficult to get your mind off the topic of baby-making. You want to have sex only to have a baby.

As each month passed the pressure of getting this right added up and took a toll on me and my husband. There was a lot of performance pressure and sex no longer was fun but a mechanical activity to make a baby. Trust me - this is the wrong'est' thing you can do.

While the doctor had clearly told us, healthy couples can take anywhere between 3 to 12 months to conceive. Also, some might conceive the first time you have unprotected sex while others might take more time, so it really depends from person to person. For us, after having tried for 2 months, the third month felt like a lot of pressure for both me and my husband.

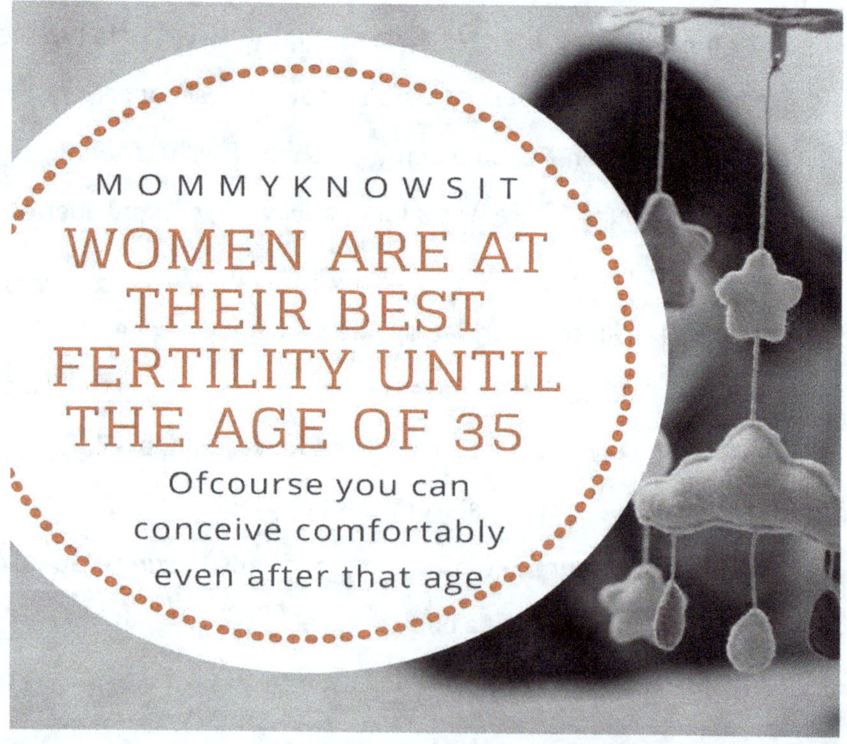

The third month probably was the worst for us. We were under so much pressure, it was all mechanical. No foreplay, nothing, hit the ground, get it done and move. I had tried everything I read about, from not showering in too hot water to keeping my legs flying up in the air to not drinking alcohol. And then came that period of the month again, my periods had become irregular since the time we started having unprotected sex. My periods were delayed that month too and out of curiosity, I tested on the 5th delayed day only to see a negative result again. I was extremely disappointed. I did not know what more to do.

My husband was supportive all through and he told me that we should not take this on as a task but maybe try and enjoy. If it happens good, if it doesn't then we can see what options we have. For me it was easier said than done but I decided to let it loose.

The fourth month I decided to take it slow, so I would not pressurize myself and my husband to have sex. I stopped monitoring the ovulation with the kit, but only started closely observing my bodily changes. When I felt like I was near to ovulation, I told my husband we should have sex alternate day and we tried to stick to it.

I was in a semi-happy state in the 4th month, trying to not think about the baby-making but to enjoy the process. While the 4th month was going on, I started to religiously do my meditation and breathing exercises mostly to keep myself sane. These exercises helped me calm down thus helping keep my mind off the baby topic. As we entered the 5th month, I was a lot better. I finally started being normal, trying to enjoy everything from my long hot showers to my occasional alcohol and still kept on with the alternate day or at least once in 3 days sex during fertile days routine on.

For those who do not know how to find out if you are ovulating or not?

Ovulation is about 12-14 days before yours periods. You can see a clearer thinner mucus (ejaculation types). Also your sex drive is high during that time

The fifth month we had sex only when we felt like, no forced acts. During the period when I felt I was ovulating, we had sex once every 2 days (I would recommend doing it every alternate day for better results). This month I had no pressure since I had decided, if it happens good, if it doesn't happen that is fine too, I had decided to go with the flow.

At the end of the fifth month, my periods got delayed like every month. I was super curious but tried to keep it calm. We live abroad and early that month we were supposed to fly to India. The day before our flight was the 7th day of the delayed period. My husband asked me not to take the pregnancy test until we land in India. While I wanted to listen to him, I thought I have only one pregnancy kit left, let me just check and boom;

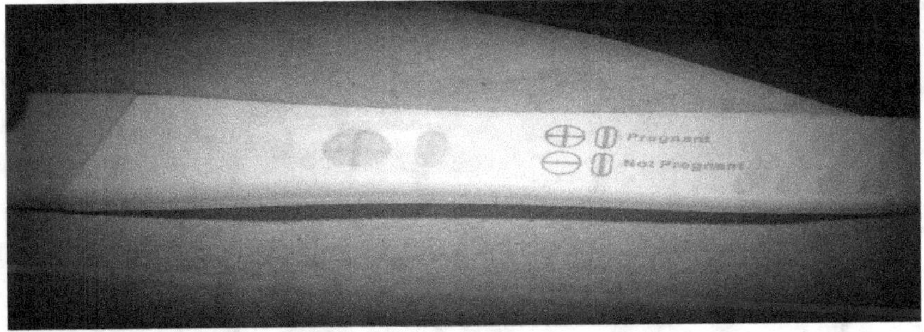

Finally, all that I was waiting for happens one day prior to my air travel.

Finally, all that I was waiting for happens one day prior to my air travel.

No one recommends traveling in the first trimester and here I was not knowing whether to be happy about the positive result or be sad that I might have to cancel my trip. We did travel the next day but more about that in the following chapters.

2. Conceiving Tips

While I have covered most of the things on conceiving in the previous chapter, I have specifically included this one to share some tips. Conceiving takes only a sperm and one of the female eggs to meet up but that can sometimes happen in a day or take months. The wait period during pregnancy isn't fun so in this chapter I'm sharing some tips that will help in getting higher positive results.

Please know that one remedy doesn't fit all, so these tips might work beautifully for some but might not for others. And it is always recommended for a couple to take gynaecologist's advice along with recommendations from this book or any other sources.

So, here's the first and the most important tip. Have sex every alternate day or with a gap of two days. Sex is the ultimate thing that will help in getting you pregnant so try to do it as much as possible. Don't make it a baby making game else it won't be fun and it would take longer to conceive. Trying different sex styles/positions, getting explorative with sex (role-playing, kinky, surprise, etc) anything that can help to elevate the mood. Making sex more fun means your mood is happier and then there are higher chances of conceiving.

I cannot stress enough on how important it is to be happy and stress-free when trying to conceive and also throughout the pregnancy. When you are trying to conceive, pregnant and post-pregnancy too, the hormones play up a lot and cause stress so it is doubly important to do things that will keep your mood lightened up. During the day at least have some time (15 - 30 minutes) to do an activity that you enjoy and can make you feel happy. It can be anything like painting or watching a comedy show or gardening or speaking to a friend. Anything that makes you happy.
Next is good sleep. Good sleep is as important as sex when trying to get pregnant. Good sleep helps keep the mind calm thus keeping stress away. Stress is the last thing you want when trying to make babies.

Along with adequate sleep, it is wonderful to keep your mind stress-free by practicing breathing exercises. Normal breathing exercises come a long way in pregnancy. You can start with simple breath in breath out, first with both nostrils, then in from one and out from other and finally in from nose and out from the mouth. These three types of breathing are mainly enough but if you have the will to do more than you can check out breathing exercises in yoga and practice those.

Breathing exercise helps cleanse your body & mind, keeps it calm and fresh. Breathing exercises also help during labour pain, so if you start practicing from the beginning, it will help you in the later phases of pregnancy too.

OVULATION

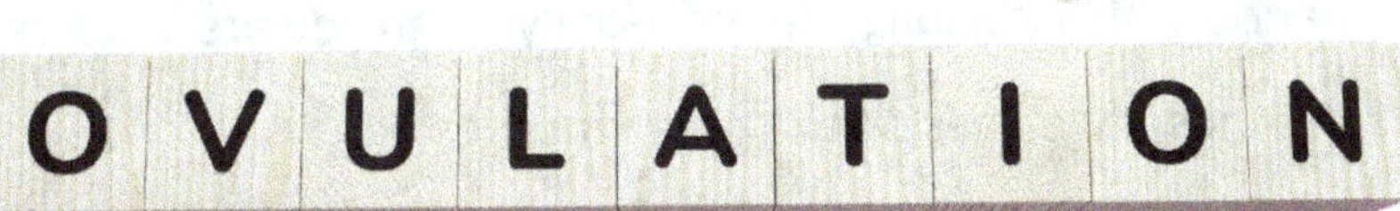

Days around ovulation are most fertile and hence when you are wanting to get pregnant, have sex maximum number of times during the ovulation period. Alternate day at minimum is must

When you decide you want to seriously try for babies, it is ideal to track your periods and ovulation days. Ovulation days are the days when females are most fertile and hence conception happens on these days. Ovulation lasts between 1 to 5 days. You get ovulation strips in the market, pee on it and it tells you whether you are ovulating or not. Sex on ovulation days is what gives you the highest chance of conception. Ensure to have sex every day or alternate day during ovulation. Once the ovulation days are passed they would occur next time only after the next period which is a long wait especially when you are desperate to get those two lines on the pregnancy test kit.

Conceiving needs a healthy body and a healthy body is achieved by having all the nutrients either through your meals or supplements. As important as the nutrients are, water is equally important. Water helps cleanse the body. Also, when conceived, the baby in your uterus is in amniotic fluid, water and protected by the placenta. Having an adequate amount of water keeps the baby infection free (this water is not plain water but staying hydrated helps regulate this level too)

Make Sex fun

=> Happy Mood

=> Quicker Conceiving

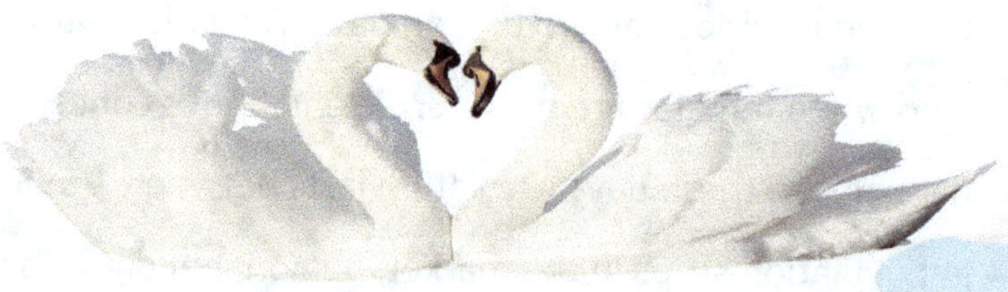

Most people start folic acid tablets once they are trying to conceive, you should continue those tablets until the end of first trimester. Based on your blood report the doctor will recommend certain supplements, ensuring to take those properly. For a healthy baby development, all nutrients are required adequately. Thyroid levels sometimes interfere with conceiving and can delay the process so try to regulate your thyroid before starting to try for a baby.

The journey of trying to get pregnant and pregnancy lead to a lot of hormonal changes. One thing that helped me greatly to keep my mood in check was good food. Being a foodie, food uplifts my mood instantly. So, if food is your love too then eat what you like and keep a happy mood. While I say eat what you like, eat everything in moderation. Excessive weight gain is not good while trying to conceive and also during pregnancy.

Last but not least, exercise to keep your body active and healthy. While eating your favourite food to keep your tummy happy is important, equally important is to exercise to keep the body healthy. If you have not been active always then don't start anything drastic when trying to conceive or when pregnant. Non-active people (sedentary lifestyle) can add walking to their routine. If exercise is not your friend then incorporating walking in your routine is an easy thing to do. Start with 15-20 minutes and you can increase it up to the point your body can do it. I had a habit of walking for an hour. I continued that until the middle of the first trimester and then my body wouldn't support it so I used to do two sets of 25minutes each. I continued walking till almost my delivery day. The only thing I kept doing was listening to my body and walking accordingly. So, if there are days when my body is feeling exhausted then I wouldn't walk or would walk less. If I am feeling ok/normal, I would walk my usual dose. If you work out regularly then you can continue that until almost the third trimester, exception of special or high-risk pregnancy.

Once you have done all of the suggested and finally notice a missed period then, take the pregnancy test after 8 days of missing your period. Use the first urine sample of the morning. If you have the habit of getting up to pee in the night, do not worry - take the sample of the early morning pee [whenever you wake up]. Check the pregnancy strip immediately, keeping it for long can give wrong results.

Some of the early symptoms of pregnancy are as follows;
- Sore Breast (painful nipples)
- Period like feeling but no periods

- Slight pain in stomach

- Tiredness and weakness

- Feverish accompanied with fever

- Nausea and uneasiness

You might experience one or all of these but please know that just experiencing these symptoms does not indicate pregnancy. So, ensure you wait at least up to 7-10 days after your missed period date and then take a pregnancy test.

The pregnancy date is calculated by considering your last period date as the first day. So essentially by the time you get to know you are pregnant, you are almost one month pregnant.

3. Being Pregnant

Being pregnant is an amazing feeling if you are trying for it, if not then it can be a terrible shocker. From chapter 1 you know me and my husband were trying to get pregnant so seeing those two lines on the pregnancy test were the awesome'est' thing I could see that morning. We contemplated whether we should travel to India or not but we decided to go ahead with our plan and pretended as if we didn't know that we were pregnant. Thankfully all went well and the pregnancy was fine.

Seeing those positive pregnancy lines brought in happiness but also tension of taking extra care about your health, food, routine and lifestyle.

As we go to the following chapters I will describe all the care/precautions to be taken to have a healthy and happy pregnancy.

While you might experience some of the symptoms mentioned in the earlier chapter like sore breasts, nausea, etc – some women experience nothing and so the initial days of pregnancy feel normal. I had so much hormonal upheaval before pregnancy that I did not feel any difference in the first few days of being pregnant. Rather, I felt like something had settled and so all the uneasiness I was having for the last few months had gone away.

An average pregnancy lasts for 40 weeks. Three trimesters are formed from the weeks. The period of time between conception to week 12 of a pregnancy is known as the first trimester. Generally, people advise against announcing pregnancy before first trimester completion and I would advise the same. The reason being that during these initial months of pregnancy, the embryo is getting attached to your uterus and at that time it is too delicate. Utmost care should be taken during this time. Not exposing yourself to X-ray or any invasive light is important. Raw meat should be avoided as it can cause infection and lead to unnecessary problems. Heavy activity or heavy movement is also to be avoided as it is a delicate phase and huge jerk can cause unwanted effects.

The first 12 weeks of a pregnancy are a time of significant physical change for a woman. Women frequently begin to worry about:

- Things to eat
- Which prenatal test kinds they ought to consider
- The potential weight increases

- Ways they can ensure the health of their infant
- Things to do

In the following chapters, you will find all the information around these questions that can be in your mind as an expectant mothers/fathers

3A. First Trimester

The first trimester of pregnancy is from Week 1 to Week 13. Normally when you take a pregnancy test you are almost 4-5 weeks pregnant, so by the time you get to know you are pregnant you are half way through the first trimester.

A lot happens during the first trimester. From the sperm being accepted in the body to the fertilized egg split up into layers of cells and implantation on the walls of your uterus. The growth is happening at a rapid pace and soon these cells start growing into the baby. Your last menstrual cycle began on the first day of your pregnancy. An egg is released 10 to 14 days later, a sperm and an egg interact, and pregnancy takes place. During the first trimester, a baby grows quickly. The organs start to grow, and the brain and spinal cord start to develop in the foetus. The first trimester is also when the baby's heart starts to beat.

In the first few weeks, arms and legs start to bud, and by the end of eight weeks, fingers and toes start to take shape. The developing baby's sex organs are formed by the end of the first trimester. The infant is now about 3 inches long and weighs about a pound.

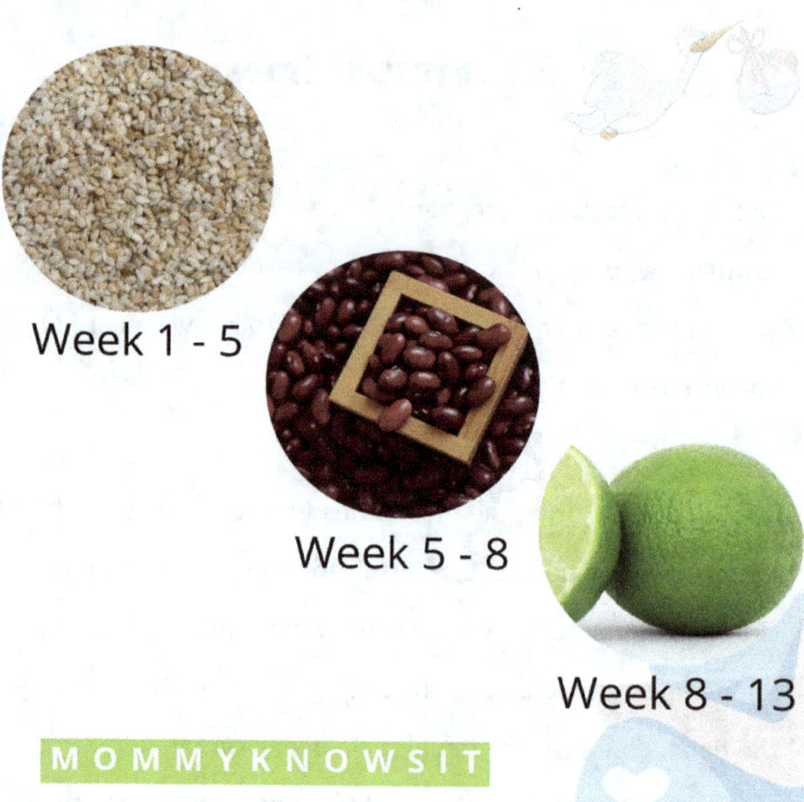

My first trimester like I mentioned started when I was finally enjoying life not worrying about getting pregnant. I missed the period and checked, it turned out to be positive. Now normally people say don't travel in the first trimester and here I was taking a 9-hour flight. I was uncertain but thought let's take the risk, what if I had not tested. Thankfully all went well, I had a safe flight and no issues with the pregnancy too. Two things that I took care of, I wore loose clothes for the journey and did not rush through anywhere. Me and my husband tried to keep the journey as comfortable and stress free as possible.

The first trimester for me was a rollercoaster of experiences. A lot of nausea, mood swings, stomach cramps, leg pain - you name it and I had it. While I took the vitamin, mineral supplements but most of the issues I tried to solve through home remedies. And trust me that is really good for your body in the long run.

The first trimester is all about taking care of little things to ensure you and the baby are safe and have good growth.

Here is a list of some quick to do's and don'ts during the first 13 weeks.

To Do:

- Take prenatal vitamins
- Continue the folic acid tablet for the first trimester or more as advised by the doctor
- Include some form of exercise – if you work out then you can continue so. If you don't workout usually then start walking on a regular basis (do it as much as your body can bear)
- Eat a rich diet – inclusive of fruits, fibre rich food, low fat form, proteins and vitamins
- Drink good amount of water

Don'ts:

- Strenuous exercises especially the ones that put pressure on the stomach
- Eating raw meat/fish/flesh
- Too much caffeine (1-2 cups of tea/coffee is ok if you have a normal pregnancy)
- Alcohol intake
- Smoking or Drugs
- Unpasteurized dairy products as they can cause unwanted bacteria to enter the body and cause issues

- Eating food that is hot for the body – shark fish, mackerel, red snapper, too many eggs

As you and the baby are getting used to being in your body and developing, this period can feel a little stressful and also your body won't feel completely normal. You might have pain/pull in the body. Also, stomach cramps can keep happening.
All throughout ensure you remain stress-free, happy, eat healthy and sleep enough.

3A1. First Trimester - Week 1 To 4

The week 1 of pregnancy is your first day of your last period. So essentially you would not know you are pregnant until that month is over and you miss your periods next month. During these 4 weeks, a lot of hormonal changes take place like mood swings, tender breast, uneasiness in the stomach (basically the uterus but until then you don't know so most people assume it to be stomach uneasiness). Some women also get spotting which is also called implantation bleeding. As the cells (baby) stick to the walls of the uterus, they shed the uterus lining causing light bleeding in the form of spotting.

Whether you have conceived or not, it is advisable to eat healthy food throughout the time you are trying to conceive. Also start taking folic acid tablets as soon as you have decided to try for a baby.

I started taking folic tablets, one tablet per day when we decided we are going to try. I continued with those tablets until the end of the first trimester.

These 4-5 weeks are quite intense, since you are waiting to know the result and curiosity and anxiety are at its peak.

During the first few weeks of pregnancy, miscarriages are common. While you cannot do anything directly to avoid it, here are some recommendations to try our best to not go through it.

- If you are trying for a baby and you get to know you are pregnant then stop smoking and drinking alcohol
- Stay active. Because you are pregnant, don't become dormant. Pregnancy is not illness and you can continue your regular activity only strenuous once should be avoided
- Eat a healthy balanced diet
- Drink enough water throughout the day

- Maintain healthy weight. Do not eat unlimitedly just because you are pregnant. Healthy mother helps give birth to a healthy baby
- Avoid food that causes heat in the body. Also, avoid eating raw food at least in the initial days of pregnancy

You should take good care of yourself during the initial days and all will be fine. You might experience a high shift of emotion, this is due to hormones playing up. If you think you have too much anxiety or are getting depressed then you should talk to your midwife/doctor. If it is usual mood swings then you can try to distract yourself by doing activities that you enjoy doing. This will distract you and also uplift your mood.

Being stress-free and happy contributes greatly to a healthy pregnancy. So, maintain your mental as well as physical health from the beginning.

3A2. First Trimester - Week 5 To 8

Week 5 is usually when you realize having missed the period and hence you would take the test. Always take the test at least 7-8 days after missing the periods. In my case, once we started having unprotected sex, my periods were thrown off cycle. I started getting a minimum 10 days delay on my period. Of course, I used to get all hopeful in those 10 days but it was always a false alarm. Also, ensure to use the first sample of the morning urine to test. Possible one wherein you haven't had any water or food before. And ensure to pee on the pregnancy test kit and check it immediately. Don't pee and leave the kit around, the evaporation/spread of pee also causes false positives that it shows two lines while it might not be positive.

So, once your pregnancy test comes out positive - the cycle of anticipation starts. I was so curious that I signed up with a couple apps, got on various websites - read extensively. Result of all that research is me writing this book...ha-ha
All through my pregnancy one thing that I enjoyed the most was knowing the size of the baby each week and its development. So, taking help from my favourite app BabyCenter, I'm going to mention those details here for you too.

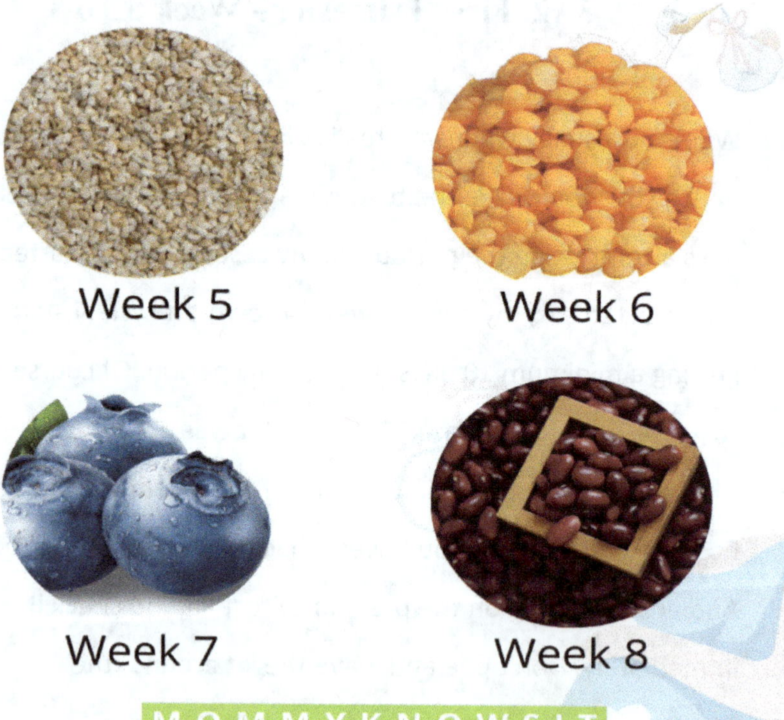

Week 5

Week 6

Week 7

Week 8

Babies get heartbeat by week 6-9 so during your second ultrasound, you should be able to hear the baby heartbeat. I was a first-time mom and hence this was a super special feeling. Due to covid my husband wasn't allowed in and I missed showing it to him terribly. So, if you are allowed to take your husband then do surely take him with you for this scan. The first scan happens at week 5/6 when you first get to know you are pregnant. It is mainly done, just to verify if you are really pregnant. If a baby heartbeat is present at this scan, then the immediate next scan is not needed. If the baby heartbeat was not heard at this scan (usually it happens at 5-8 weeks) then they might call you for a scan again at 7/8 weeks. Once the baby's heartbeat has started, you have crossed one milestone of the baby growth in pregnancy. While from six weeks, a heartbeat is usually heard, by the end of week 12, your baby's bones, muscles and all the organs of the body are formed. At this point, your baby looks like a tiny human being and is now called a foetus.

The umbilical cord is also formed during this period around week 7-8. It is the connection between the mother and the baby, providing the baby with oxygen and nourishment. It is also used by the baby's body to dispose of waste. The mouth, nostrils, ears and eyes are some of the facial features that become more defined during this period. The lungs and digestive tract are also getting formed now.

Pregnancy causes a lot of changes to the cervix. One of the major things is the mucus plug. The mucus plug is developed in the early weeks and by week 7-8, the mucus plug seals the uterus. This is how the baby is protected from any infection. Now as weeks progress the baby will grow in the uterus. The baby will be surrounded by amniotic liquid and water as they call it. This remains inside the uterus due to the mucus plug. As your pregnancy comes to an end, the mucus plug falls off and that is the start of labour. More about this in the third last chapter where I have described the entire labour process.

I started getting quite a bit of morning sickness in the first trimester - mainly from week 5. And please know that morning sickness does not just stay in the morning, it stays throughout the day. I had it for all of my first trimester.

As I progressed through the weeks, the intensity of it kept increasing.

What helped me to keep the nausea down were some Indian remedies (Ghar ke nuske) - like having buttermilk, lassi (thick yogurt with sugar), Lemon Water (Nimbu Paani), Raw Mango Juice in Jaggery (Aam Panna), coconut water and cold milk. The gynaecologist or midwife does give you a tablet for nausea but I tried to avoid tablets as much as possible and relied on natural remedies.

Initially the nausea was bearable so I randomly did stuff but as the intensity increased I followed the following routine.

- Morning on waking up - 2 cup of hot water followed by coconut water
- Breakfast - Not fixed, anything from bread butter, bread jam, bread omelette, indian breakfast items (poha or upma)
- 15-20 minutes prior to lunch - a glass of buttermilk. If the nausea was high some days, I used to have buttermilk through the meal [Do not add too much salt in the buttermilk, as it can cause other side effects like itching. If you have rock salt/black salt - use that]
- Evening around 5-6PM - a glass of Aam Panna (Raw mango juice with jaggery) or Lemon juice with little salt (nimbu pani)
- Had an Indian digestive tablet called hajmola 15-20 minutes before dinner
- Dinner
- Half cup cold milk before sleeping

This routine greatly helped me survive the nausea and for me to have meals. With the nausea, I had no urge to eat and surely no cravings whatsoever.

Do not add too much salt/sugar while making the suggested drinks. Salt - possibly use black salt and that too in moderation. Sugar - You can use jaggery but if you have to use sugar, use in moderation.

Also, on days when you don't feel as nauseated, try to avoid having drinks with salt/sugar also the hajmola. Hajmola mainly helps temporarily to remove the nauseated feeling and in my case, it helped me feel normal for a bit thus helping me to eat. Along with all these, ensure to stay hydrated by having a good amount of water intake through the day.

During this time your sex drive can be high and you can have the urge to have sex. There is no scientific proof which says you shouldn't have sex in the first trimester but I kept away from it. I felt the first trimester is quite tender as the baby is just taking grips in the uterus and hence I did not want any risk of spotting, etc and so I stayed away from it but if you are not the high-risk pregnancy type then you can indulge in sex or in some self-pleasure activity to satisfy the urge.

By week 8 your little bean is really the size of a bean with all vital

organs developed.

3A3. First Trimester - Week 9 To 13

The initial days of pregnancy are funny since you don't feel much but only nausea. And some days if you don't have nausea you get scared whether you are really pregnant or not. By week 9, your little bub has become the size of an olive.

Your boobs start becoming tender by the day and can be quite painful sometimes. By this time, you start wondering how I should sleep, should I sleep on my sides or on the back. Please know that the baby is safe in your womb and has multiple layers of skin/fat/protection so however you sleep you can't really harm the baby at this stage. I was lucky to get a good gynaecologist in India, she had told me I can even sleep on my tummy. She said you can't really harm the baby by sleeping and as you grow through the pregnancy there are certain positions you won't be able to sleep in, so the baby makes sure it doesn't allow you any position that you can hurt it in. So, she recommended that I just listen to my body and act accordingly. I truly did that through the pregnancy and felt super lucky to deliver a healthy baby at the end of it all.

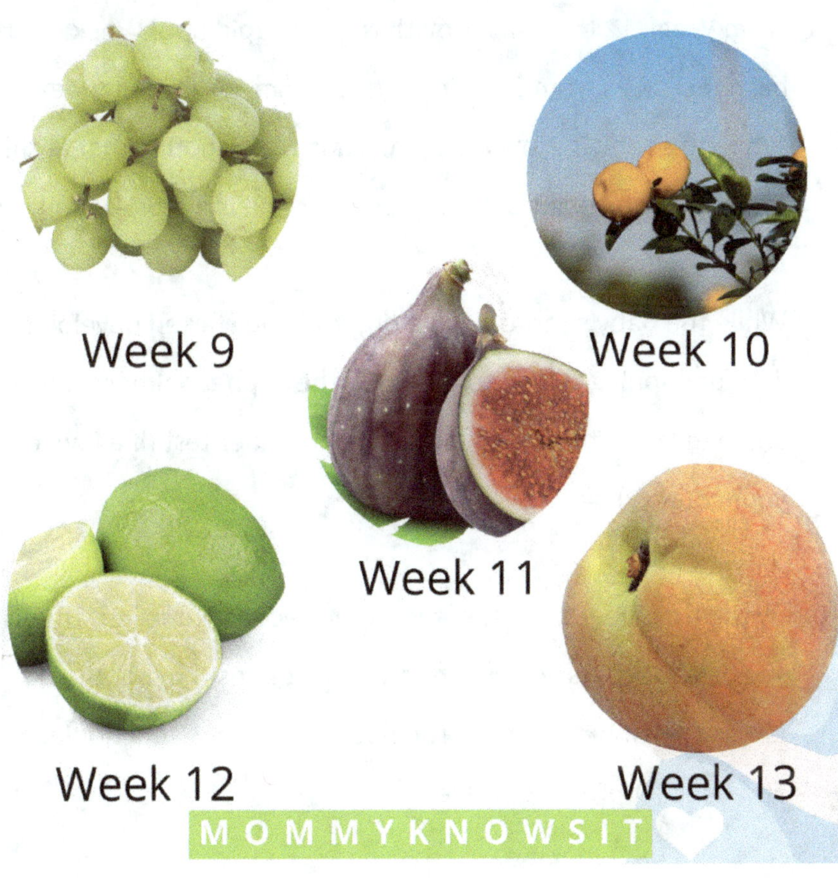

Week 9

Week 10

Week 11

Week 12

Week 13

As you near the end of the first trimester most of the morning sickness symptoms go away and you start feeling pregnant by the tummy now - as in you would feel some movement in the tummy making you feel pregnant. For some women there is a slight bulge in the tummy by this time. I am on the heavier side of weight and hence did not really see any bulge until mid-second trimester.

From Week 12 the baby growth is quite rapid until Week 20. The baby increases from 5 cm to almost 20 cm in these few weeks. While the baby is growing rapidly, it is worth noting that at this stage the baby head is the biggest part and is almost half of the body length.
While the baby's reproductive organs have started developing and functioning but up to week 14, they appear almost similar and hence it is then that you take the gender test (if allowed in your country).

By the time your body is entering the second trimester, the baby has developed its vocal cords and now opens the mouth and drinks the amniotic liquid. The baby kidneys are functioning now and hence it produces urine.

While the baby is growing, your body is also adapting to this new way of being. Your blood flow is increased quite a bit, also the oil glands secrete additional oil, all of which leads to a glowing skin. Some women also start getting pregnancy acne. But do not worry. Most of the pregnancy related things go away after you deliver the baby. So just enjoy the phase and the baby growth.

During the first trimester, you might undergo a pregnancy marker test, which many refer to as the **first-trimester screening**, it involves a blood sample along with a unique ultrasound known as the **nuchal translucency (NT) scan**. This test is usually done for moms to be above the age of 30 but sometimes for others too. Depends on if your gynaecologist/midwife feels the need for it. It combines a blood test measuring specific pregnancy hormones with a specialized ultrasound called an NT scan, which measures the fluid space at the back of the baby's neck. A thicker fluid measurement or unusual hormone levels can indicate a higher risk for physical or chromosomal variations. Ultimately, the test combines these measurements with your age to calculate a personalized risk score (Low, Intermediate, or High risk) for conditions like Down syndrome, letting you know if further diagnostic testing is recommended.

3B: Second Trimester

Once you cross the first trimester safely, the chances of miscarriage are lesser and hence less stress for the expectant mother. The second trimester is the fun trimester. The nausea/morning sickness/uneasiness is all gone. You are free to satisfy that food craving finally and most importantly you start to feel the baby slightly. Also, your tummy starts growing so you feel bodily pregnant too.

This was the trimester I could really enjoy being in India. Since the time I had arrived I was unable to eat even my favourite food due to nausea. I tried to make the most of my mom's food and all my favourite delicacies.

Things to do in the wonderful second trimester

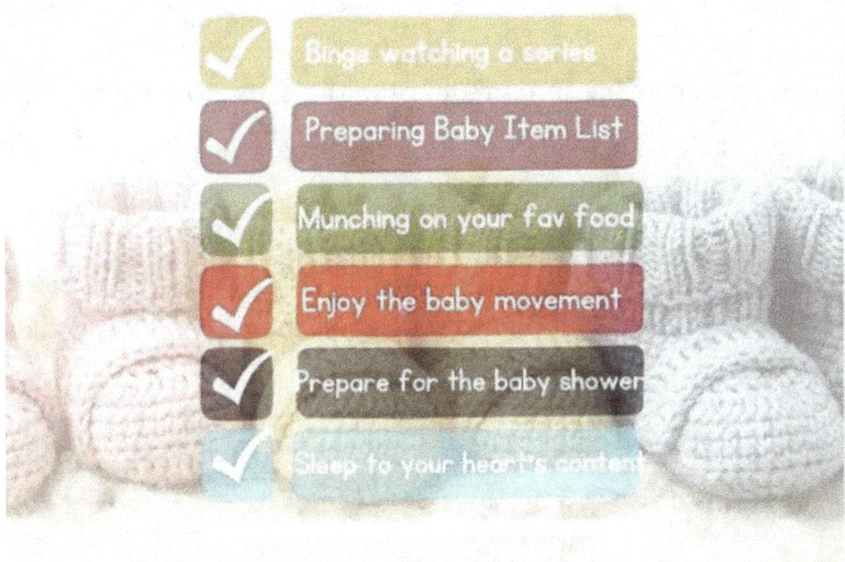

The second trimester is the safest trimester, so you can work out a fair bit in these 3 months. But please keep in mind that if you haven't worked out before pregnancy do not start anything now. In those cases, just add walks to your daily routine. I normally work out a bit but I had stopped some time before pregnancy. I did not want to do anything drastic so I continued my walking sessions - in the first trimester I started with 20 minutes each day and increased it to 60 minutes a day. During the second trimester, I went on for 90 minutes a day. One key thing that helped me ensure I wasn't overdoing was listening to my body. If I felt tired/exhausted, I took a break. Sometimes I split the walking up in 3-4 sessions of 20-30 minutes each.

As you enter the second trimester, the baby growth is happening at a rapid pace. And every time you have your check, you would hear some new movement by the baby. The baby is now able to feel their hands, fingers and hence knows to put those hands in their mouth. My boy loved sucking his thumb when in my tummy. For almost 3 of our scans we saw him sucking on his hand/thumb. It is funny and cute to see this little human doing activities that we humans do.

While the second trimester is the fun trimester, it also is the trimester where the baby develops and gets to all the usual human functioning so internally a lot of changes are happening to the mother's body. Some women develop regular headaches or dry skin or itchiness or forgetfulness. But like I have mentioned earlier you should remember that all this is temporary. Once the baby is out, you will have your normal body back – not immediately but in some time. And all these problems that have developed during pregnancy will disappear.

This is the trimester when all the blood tests for gestational diabetes, thyroid and other ailments are done. Also, if you are not in India then this is the trimester you get to know the baby gender. So, while fun, this trimester is also an important one.

This is your time to enjoy to-be-mommy

MommyKnowsIt

3B1. Second Trimester - Week 14 To 18

The first trimester can be a little taxing given the nausea, bodily and mental changes, so the second trimester feels like a breeze of fresh air. The baby is growing fast and now it starts to make slight movements. Your baby's ovaries or testes are developing during this time and soon the baby will show a tiny willy or penis.

This trimester is lighter on the body as the body has now gotten used to having the baby inside so mostly you will have no morning sickness, also the body doesn't ache as much as it used to. So, it is time to satisfy all the cravings but do keep in mind that you need to have everything in balance.

Pregnancy puts the hormones for a toss and hence too much random eating can cause unnecessary issues. I love Mumbai chat, sea food and Indian Chinese but my doctor had told me to stay away from Indian Chinese as they add MSG which is not good for health even in normal circumstances. To satisfy my craving, I ate everything apart from Chinese in moderation. Chinese food, I only had a couple spoons just to satisfy my craving.

And most importantly, I tried to make everything at home so I tried to keep it as hygienic as

possible, also wherever possible I added veggies to keep my nutrient count high.

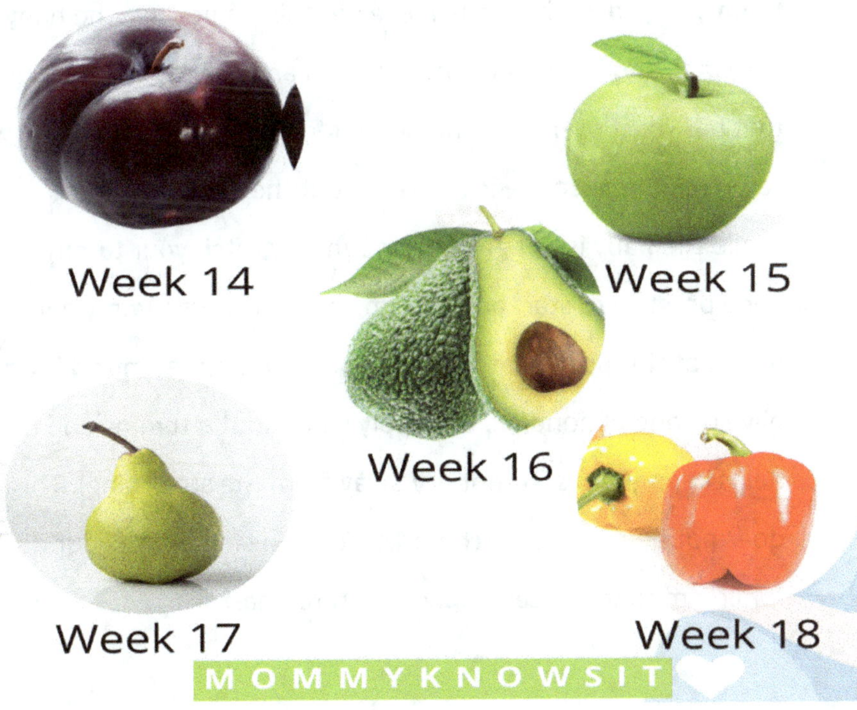

Ensure you eat as much as your body needs, don't eat more just because you are pregnant or don't eat less to avoid weight gain. If you maintain a healthy weight through the pregnancy, all your pregnancy weight will go away by the time your baby turns 2-3 months. Do not fall for the myth of eating for 2 people because you are pregnant. If you need to eat for two people, your body will give you hunger signals. Eat only as much as needed.

The baby is growing from being the size of a small lemon to a bell pepper (capsicum) by week 18. As a mother it is fun to imagine the baby growing and to start feeling your tummy a little. Your tummy wouldn't show much even at this point since the baby is still small and it is mainly the placenta and the water in the uterus that has most of the weight. Some females do show up early while some take time so do not worry about the tummy size.
While the baby is not grown enough to stretch your tummy, it is a good practice to start applying some oil on your tummy and breast at this point. I used coconut oil, sometimes mixed it with olive oil and almond oil. But applying oil to the tummy and boobs helps keep them soft (not dry away from the stretching). This does not help with stretchmarks. You can check with your doctor for cream that you can apply for stretchmarks.

During this time, chances of getting urinal infection are quite high. If you experience any burning sensation, itching down there, see your doctor and get ointment to get it fixed. Vaginal infection is pretty common during pregnancy so watch out for symptoms and get it addressed immediately. Having an infection in the vagina for too long is not good for the baby.

Any time during your pregnancy if you experience itching on your hands (especially palm) or feet, then speak to your doctor immediately. These are signs of liver issue which generally occurs later in pregnancy (third trimester) however for some women, it might occur earlier too. I had this kind of itching on my body and my doctor got me to do the Liver Function Test. All came out fine and it turned out that my salt intake had increased and hence the itching. My doctor prescribed some ointments which helped curb the itching, in the meanwhile I reduced my salt intake and I was back to normal. Also, when the itching occurs for whatever reason – applying ghee (Indian clarified butter) can help relieve the itching for a bit.

By the end of week 18, your baby has developed hearing and can hear your voice slightly. The baby also starts feeling/seeing light. Your baby starts to get light hiccups and the count of hiccups increases as you progress in the pregnancy. It is the little rhythmic flutters you feel in your tummy, it is said that hiccups are a sign of good health of the baby so don't worry if you experience those flutters in your tummy.

3B2. Second Trimester - Week 19 To 23

By this time, you start feeling completely pregnant and might have experienced the baby move too. You'll have a scan, known as the 'foetal anomaly scan' between 18 and 21 weeks. The reason for this scan is to check the growth and development of your baby. Along with this, you will go for the NIPT scan. It is done any time before week 21. The NIPT is a screening test in which a blood sample from a pregnant woman is tested. The blood sample is tested in a laboratory. If this screening test shows that the baby may have Down syndrome, Edwards' syndrome or Patau's syndrome, follow-up diagnostic testing is needed, just to be sure.

At this scan, the sonographer can tell the baby gender (might not happen if you are in India or countries where gender reveal is not allowed).

Your baby is growing fast and gaining weight week by week but they don't gain enough until the final weeks to make it super heavy for you. At this point due to the increased blood flow, your body might feel warmer. Wear loose clothes and keep yourself hydrated with good water intake. This period also marks the start of pregnancy pigmentation. You can get either white or dark patches on your skin. It is normal in pregnancy and goes away gradually post-delivery.

Some women might see a dark line appearing on the belly. This is called a linea nigra and goes away on its own post-delivery. It appears around week 20.

Regular mediation, breathing exercises help greatly in keeping the mental issues under check.

MommyKnowsIt

Certain supplements conflict
with each other so check and
take with adequate gap to
ensure proper absorption

Example:

Calcium & Magnesium can't be taken together

Vitamin C and B 12 not be taken together

It is not uncommon to see mood swings or mental anxiety all
through pregnancy. If you notice any such things, ensure to speak
to your doctor. Regular mediation, breathing exercises help
greatly in keeping the mental issues under check. Breathing
exercises are needed to ease yourself out during labour so it is a

good idea to start practicing breathing from this time of the pregnancy itself.

As the baby grows, it pulls nutrients from the mother's body. While most people might recommend you to increase your food intake, only increase food intake if you feel the need for it. Do not eat extra just because you are pregnant. Your body demands extra if you need it. I literally never increased my food intake and had a completely healthy baby (my baby was 9 lb at birth).

Around this time of pregnancy, I started getting leg cramps at night. It is called restless leg syndrome wherein your legs feel uneasy. It started at week 20-21 and it went on till almost delivery and was there for a bit even post-delivery. While you can't completely get rid of it, including magnesium supplements help big time with it. You can either take a magnesium tablet directly or have a magnesium bath. Both are equally effective. Also, ensure to take calcium supplements. They help with leg syndrome but also are good since the baby is pulling calcium from your body to build its bones so it is a good idea to refill your supply.

3B3. Second Trimester - Week 24 To 27

The second trimester as per me is the best trimester of the whole pregnancy. While the baby is growing and you get to experience all the fun things like the baby movement, etc – you do not feel any other issues (generally). The Gestational diabetes test is done during this period. During pregnancy as the hormones are playing around, some women experience a temporary type of diabetes – it is called gestational diabetes. It occurs during pregnancy and mainly goes off once you have delivered the baby. To check if a pregnant woman is suffering from it, the glucose test is done. You have to go in for an empty stomach glucose test. They ask you to drink a glass of glucose water (the hospital/laboratory provides it.). Once you drink the liquid, they draw the blood. The blood is tested three times– each time in a gap of 45-60 minutes and you are supposed to drink a little more glucose every time. Once all the blood tests are done, the results come out in a day or two. The results indicate whether you have gestational diabetes or not. If you do, the doctor will advise a special diet to keep it under control. Some expectant mothers also need to take medicine/insulin to keep the sugar levels under control. Usually females who get gestational diabetes have to go through C-section for delivery. Nutritional food, good water intake, exercises and a stress-free mind can help keep gestational diabetes away.

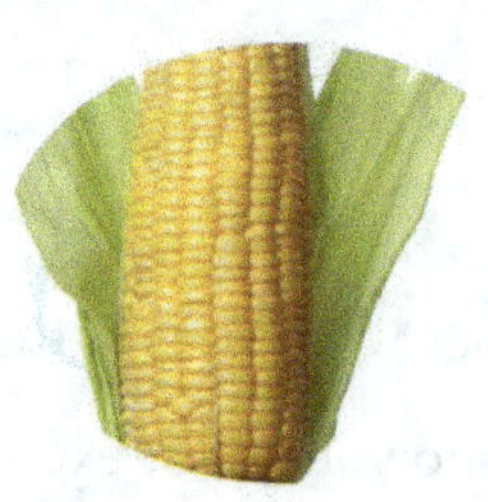

Corn @Week 24

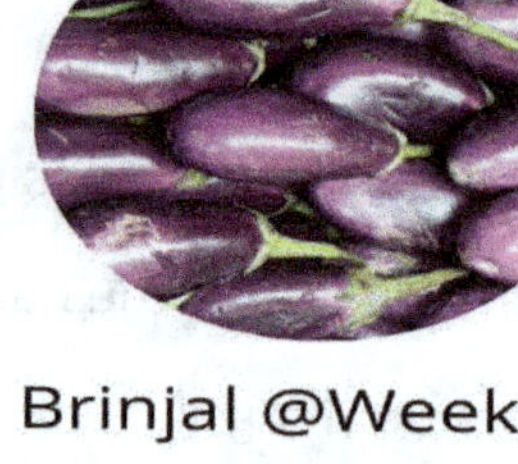

Brinjal @Week 25

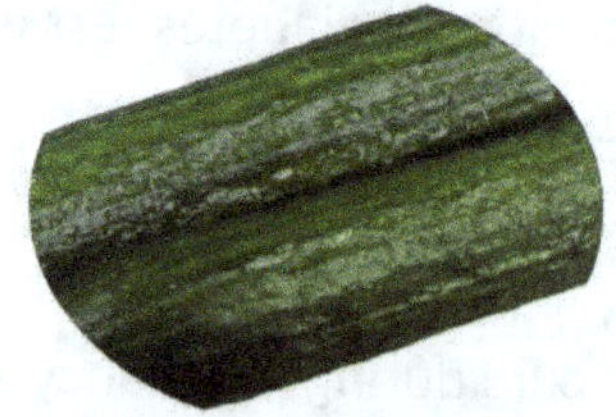

Cucumber @Week 26

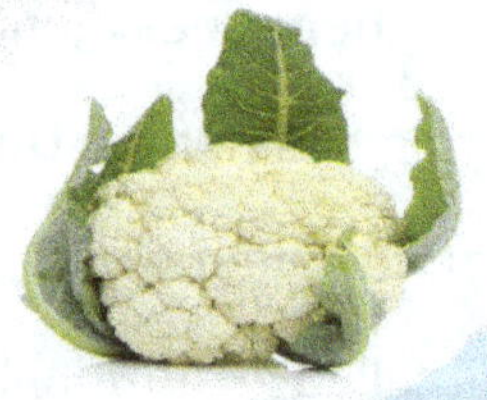

Cauliflower @Week 27

The baby bump is growing each day, in some women it grows to be huge while in some it remains petite. My bump did not show much until I entered the third trimester. The baby bump is not directly proportional to the baby size so don't worry of having a tiny baby if your bump isn't showing up much or of having a big baby if you have a big bump. As long as your scans are fine and you are experiencing all that you need to, you are good and the baby is fine!

Some women start experiencing vaginal discharge at this point. It is important to maintain hygiene down there so ensure you clean your vagina with water regularly. If you experience any itching, irritation then do see the doctor – you do not want to risk having an infection at this point.

Keep a healthy diet. Also, continue to take the supplements given by your doctor regularly. Make sure your diet is rich in calcium as calcium is needed for the baby's bone development. Calcium is found in dairy products, oranges, nuts, pulses and broccoli. You should also be taking 10mcg of vitamin D a day in pregnancy, which helps with calcium absorption.

During this period, you might start to feel some stretches in the stomach, slight stomach ache as well. It is nothing to worry about, as the baby is growing, it is making space for itself. But do contact your doctor if stomach pain is accompanied with bleeding/spotting or burning sensation while peeing.

You will have a final blood test before entering the third trimester. This blood test mainly is to check your iron levels. To ensure your iron levels are right and enough for your body to go through the intense baby birth process [might not be done if you have no iron deficiency history]. If there is any deficiency found, then your doctor/midwife will prescribe iron supplements. When you start taking Iron supplements remember your poop starts to come out as black, so don't get scared if you see black poop. Iron tablets are also known to induce nausea, constipation and overall sick feeling. If you experience any of these then speak to your doctor/midwife so that they can provide an alternative. Taking the iron tablets in the first half of the day (after breakfast) helped me keep the nausea down. You should see which time to take the tablet that works for you best and stick to it.

3C. Third Trimester

The third trimester was my scariest trimester. After a very fun second trimester, I did not expect it to be problematic again. The third trimester started with me experiencing morning sickness again but this time in the form of heartburn. And this burning sensation in the throat was terrible - I would crave to eat things but I couldn't really eat anything. Having non-spicy food, home remedies for nausea - nothing really helped fix the problem. I would get temporary relief but the problem was back in an hour.

A few weeks into the trimester the heartburn problem increased so much that I couldn't sleep at night. I had to sit and sleep through the night.

Sleeping during this time felt like a punishment but the pregnancy pillow helped me quite a bit. It helped to elevate my body slightly which helped with the heartburn also at this point your tummy is a lot heavier so you can't easily turn sides. The pregnancy pillow helps to support the tummy thus giving you a little comfort while sleeping.

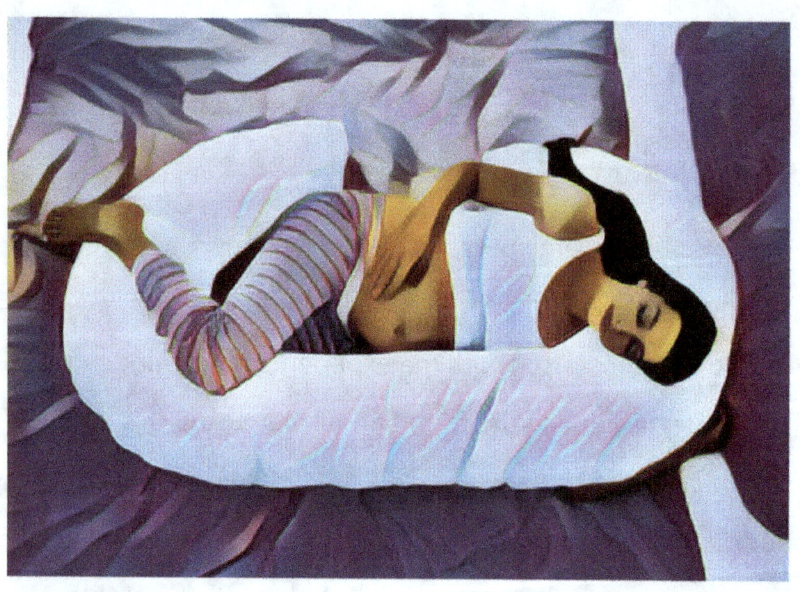

Also, by this time your tummy is quite heavy so there is a lot of pressure on your bladder causing frequent urination. Due to that you can't really sleep long hours and it adds to your tiredness. You might also experience gum bleeding. And constipation at this point is natural. Add loads of fibre to your diet so that you can keep constipation under control.

In the first and second trimester the growth of the baby is at a certain rate but the baby starts growing rapidly as you land in the third trimester. I had gained about 3-5kgs by the second trimester and I gained almost 7 kgs in the third trimester alone.

While the third trimester is tricky, I would strongly recommend you enjoy your time as much as possible. Take as much rest as possible and do everything that you need to, to feel happy. Once the baby is here, life gets very busy so enjoy this time while it is there.

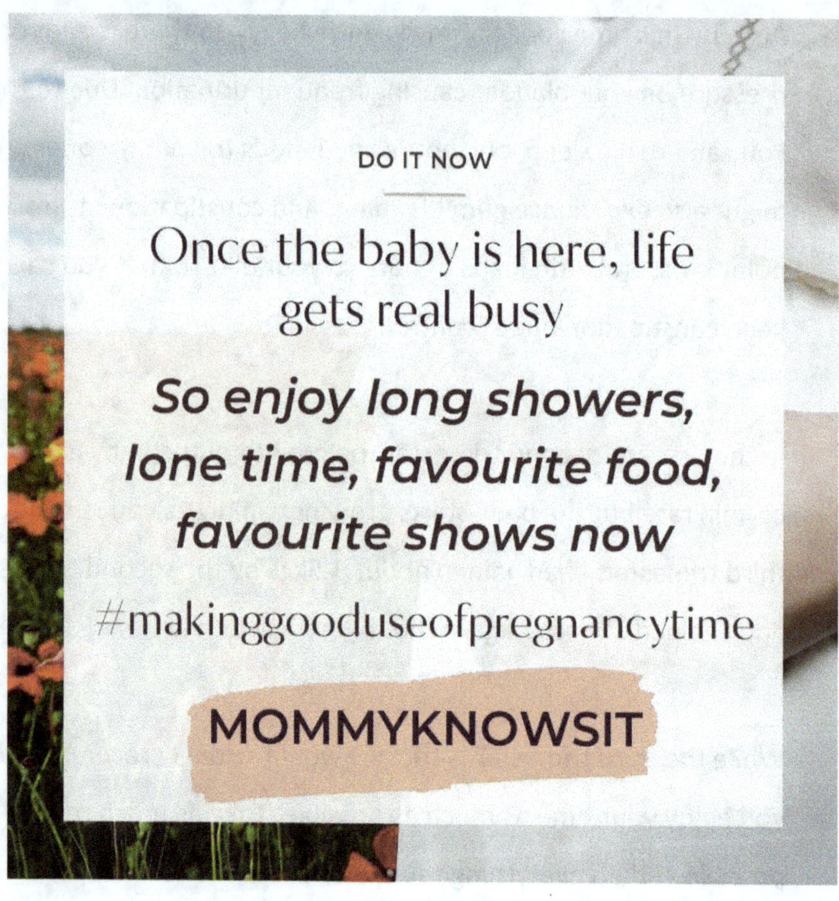

It is ideal to keep all your baby stuff ready before you hit the third trimester. As the baby grows rapidly in the third trimester, you would feel tired most of the time and might find it hard to get work done. So, whether it is getting the baby clothes, diapers or other things that the baby might need, best to do it during the second trimester or early third trimester.

3C1. Third Trimester - Week 28 To 32

The baby and the womb in general have been growing rapidly and pushing your stomach parts away to make space for themselves. Feeling acidic, experiencing heartburn and tiredness are all normal. The baby is rapidly growing and also moving around in the womb. So now you should experience a regular stream of movement by the baby. You might also note a certain pattern like my baby used to be super active in the night and lazy during the day 😄 ensuring mamma doesn't sleep and is getting ready for when he/she is out.

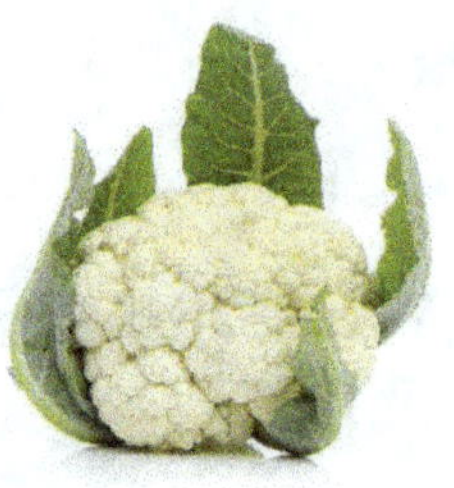

Cauliflower @Week 28

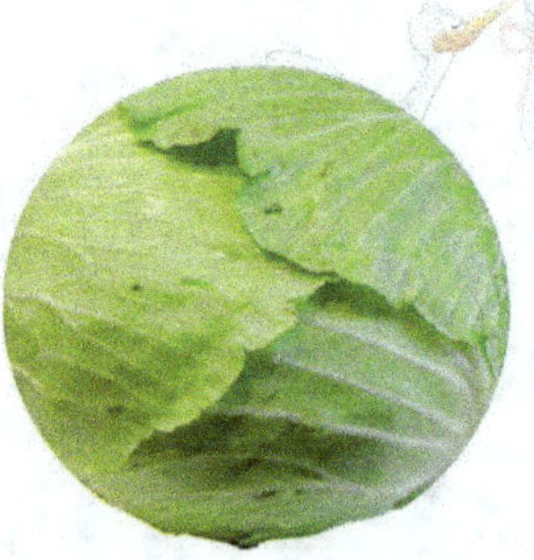

Cabbage @Week 29

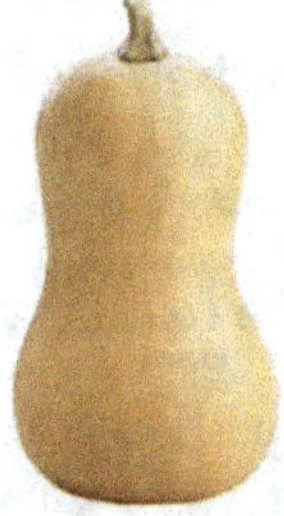

Buttersquash@Week 30

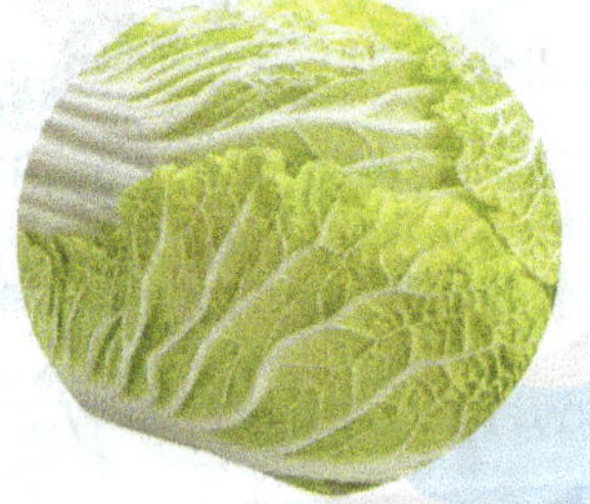

Large cabbage @Week 31/32

Noting baby movement is critical in the third trimester. Any time you feel that the baby is not moving for quite some time, you should inform your doctor or midwife. Science says babies move about 30 times each hour - while I did not ever count it to be thirty and no one can because the baby moves in the womb where there is placenta and the water which reduces the movement impact. Thus, you don't really feel each of the baby movements but in general you should be alert to know if the baby is moving. Also notice the baby movement pattern and see if it is being followed.

During my third trimester, it was twice that I felt no baby movement. I tried all the tricks like drinking cold water, warm shower, lying on one side, loud sound near my tummy and bright light (spotlight) on the tummy but nothing seemed to make the baby move so I called the midwife/doctor. She called me to the clinic, did a sonography and the baby was fine. They also kept monitoring for half an hour, it notes the baby heart beat and movement. While it is odd to keep complaining about the same thing again and again to the midwife/doctor but in this case (baby movement), I would say no shame and do it as many times as you need. It is critical and no baby movement can be a dangerous sign. My midwife told me that it is fine if it is a false alarm but better to get it checked every time rather than being sorry later. I cannot agree more - the baby is too precious to lose so keep a close eye on the baby movement.

**From the mid-second trimester you might start experiencing baby movement - on & off
Baby movement becomes very evident in the third trimester and you must monitor it to ensure the baby is moving.**

If in the third trimester you notice no baby movement, inform your doctor/midwife immediately

My third trimester started with heartburn which kept increasing through the cycle. As the baby grows, it starts making space for itself thus cramping your organs mainly your digestive system which causes indigestion, acidity and other digestive issues. Having fibre rich food during this time greatly helps to keep the constipation under check. In my case, the heartburn was so stubborn that no remedy/medicine was helping. I kept trying different things and it would work for a day or two and then no effect. Below is a brief summary of all that I tried to help curb the heartburn and to make my body accept some food. Please note that some of the things mentioned below like having cola are not really a healthy practice but that is what helped me get some food in my system so I did. You should check and see what works for you and also do things in consultation with your midwife/doctor so that you don't put yourself and the baby at risk.

- While it is ideal to get your hospital bag ready by the end of the second trimester, it is also ok to do it in the first/second lap of the third trimester. Here are some suggestions for what to add in the hospital bag;
- Comfortable clothes & Slip on - Comfy clothes are a must postpartum. Avoid anything too restrictive (other than a supportive nursing bra) and keep in mind a few options in case of a C-section. Carry a comfortable slip on for you to wear for moving around in the hospital room. Ensure they are loose since you might have swollen feet.
- Baby clothes, cap, car seat, milk bottle – Carry all of the baby stuff that is needed to get the baby safely home

- A robe - A comfortable robe is one of the best postpartum clothing items out there. It's useful if you have a vaginal delivery or a C-section.
- Toiletries – Carry your toothbrush, toothpaste, hairbrush, deodorant, hair ties.
- Your birth plan – If you have a birth plan, keep it handy so that you can share it with the hospital or relevant personnel
- Cell phone charger and a long cord/extension - Hospital beds are usually far from the electrical outlet. And you surely want your phone charged to take all the congratulations calls.
- Snacks and drinks – Pack good amount of energy drink, energy bars and anything that you like to eat and gives you strength
- Adult diapers and other postpartum care products – The hospital has a supply of all this but best to have it in your bag too.

3C2. Third Trimester - Week 33 To 37

As you reach this second lap of the third trimester, you must have grown quite a bit. Even those like me who did not show a tummy before will start showing up quite evidently now.

I was with a normal tummy (not seen much) until my 5th month. My tummy started growing a bit as I entered the 6th month and then was growing like crazy in the final trimester. And we could see it visibly with the tummy getting big and I was getting more uncomfortable internally with each passing day.

The tummy was growing and you could now see the baby moving from the top as well. Ofcourse, the mother experiences a lot of internal movements at this point but even from outside you can see slight movement of the baby.

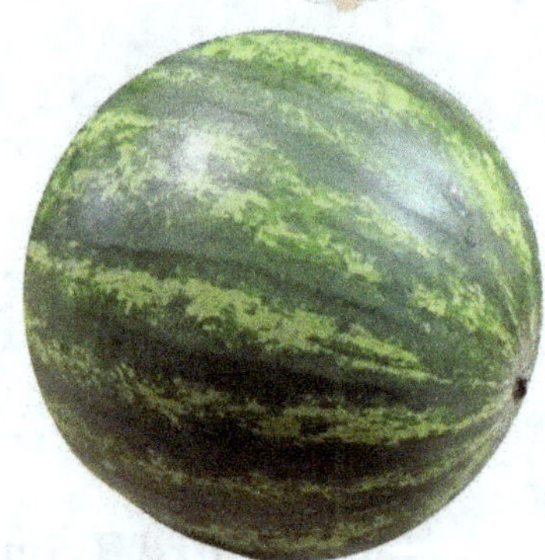

Watermelon @Week 35+

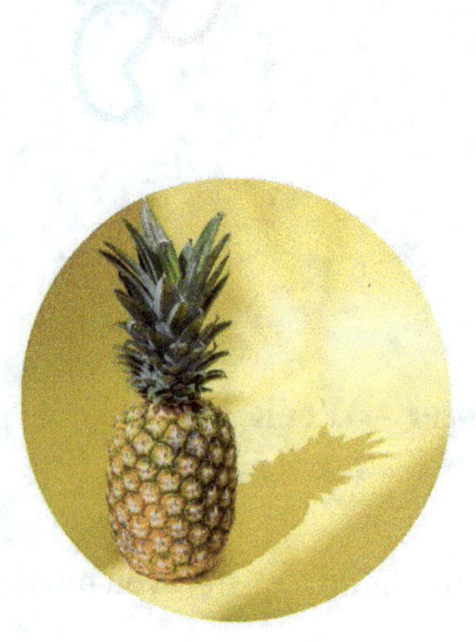

Pineapple @Week 33/34

As the baby was growing fast, it was pushing my organs left right centre to make space for itself and so I would feel sudden pain here and there. Also, my bladder was completely pressed, so I had the urge to pee every now and then. Night sleeps included at least 3-4 toilet breaks at minimum. And even more if the heartburn doesn't let you sleep.

When the tummy starts growing and you start putting on weight, it becomes tricky to look what's ahead and hence walking can get difficult. Also, your feet can hurt due to this additional weight. Though you might have all sorts of pain, try to keep an active lifestyle. I continued walking for about 60 mins in laps of 2 sets (25-30 mins in one go). Apart from this I did all my house chores until the last day (delivery day). Active lifestyle really helped me to get back on my feet quickly in-spite of an unplanned and sudden C-section. Please take guidance from your healthcare provider if you have high risk pregnancy or gestational diabetes. Mine was a normal pregnancy hence I could do all of this but high risk or gestational diabetes cases need special care.

As you are in the final days of the third trimester, the wait to see the baby gets unbearable. Each day feels too long to pass and your urge to hold your baby gets stronger.

With all the additional weight, your body starts getting tired too soon. Your stamina levels are really low and a job that you could have done in one go might need multiple iterations. Though I continued to do all house chores until the day of delivery, my stamina was low and I had to take frequent breaks.

3C3. Third Trimester - Week 38 To 42

Coming to this week feels like almost delivery time. And as we get closer to the day, the wait becomes unbearable. You get desperate to see your baby, feel your piece of heart - so each day feels like a burden. By this week, the baby development has completed and any delivery after week 38 is safe and considered a full pregnancy term.

As I entered the 38th week, I was too tired with the heartburn which did not let me eat anything, sleep properly - I was tired and worn out full time. With that, I was also desperate to see my sweetheart.

From week 37 I started doing some of the natural induction practices. I will list down all the natural induction practices and also mention which one I tried. But I must tell you, my baby loved being in the womb and was not ready to come out soon. So, while I tried to do the natural induction, my baby did not move/come out.

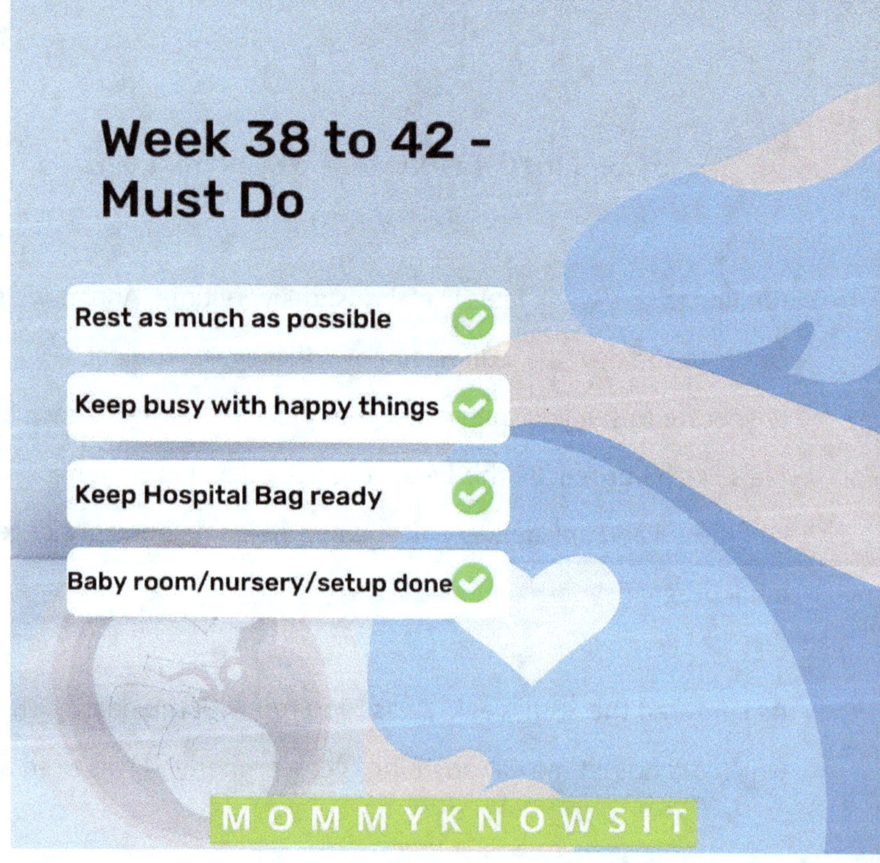

Self-induction techniques:

- Eat dates (I was eating dates since I entered third trimester - they say it helps soften the cervix thus helping in natural birth)
- Drink chamomile tea (Did not work to induce labour but it was really calming drinking it)
- Nipple stimulation (You kind of press the nipple as if the baby is breastfeeding, sometimes you might get little droplets - I did not get anything)
- Walking (I was doing that throughout the pregnancy)
- Eat spicy food (I had severe heartburn, I couldn't imagine having spicy food)
- Have sex (I was here with a heavy tummy, sleepless nights, tired - sex is the last thing I wanted to do - so I did not do it)
- Do things that make you happy (Watch favourite show, go out with friends, do anything that will make you happy internally)
- Acupuncture session (I did not do it, but people say it helps)
- Drinking castor oil - it isn't safe (I did not do it and won't recommend it)

I was waiting for the baby to arrive and each day would wake up hoping I would feel labour pain at least today. These last four weeks I tried to take as much rest as possible. I also enjoyed relaxing and watching some of my favourite movies and shows. And I would recommend everyone to do that. Once the baby arrives, life is completely different and gets too busy. So, enjoy relaxing and taking as much rest as possible when pregnant.

4. Bundle of Joy Is Here (Delivery)

As you are going through each pregnancy week your eagerness to meet your baby is increasing. You wonder what would it look like, would it be a doll or a prince, will the baby look like me or my partner, the questions in your mind are endless. When the pregnancy began you could feel really nothing but today you feel its heartbeat, its movement and now you have a connection with this baby that you haven't seen.

I was desperately waiting for my baby's arrival but my baby was enjoying being in quite a bit. After having tried almost all the natural self-induction things, I left it to happen on its own. Finally, after 41 weeks and 5 days, the water broke and the mucus plug was out.

It was an Indian festival [Diwali day - Dhanteras], I cleaned the whole house and decorated it. I'm a sucker for decoration and lights. I was extremely happy that the house was lit up ♥ ▢, I ordered sweets and was preparing for doing a small ceremony in the evening. By mid-afternoon I started getting some pain in my tummy. It was not the usual pain but I thought it was the baby getting bigger or moving, so I ignored it.

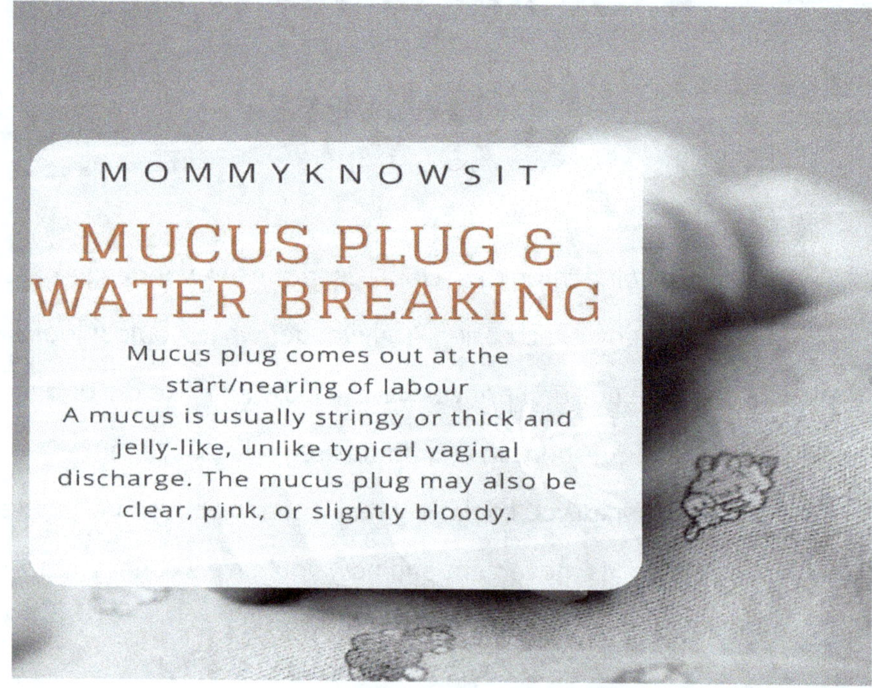

At about 6 PM when I was speaking to my mom I felt a gush of water, an uncontrollable splash, so I rushed to the toilet. I realized my water broke, so I immediately put up a sanitary pad. I called my midwife to inform about it. She asked me to monitor and to keep her informed. I could feel losing the mucus plug, it is a bloody slimy semi liquid thing, it is like the stop point at the vagina. Once it comes out, the water in the vagina comes out.

WATER BREAKING

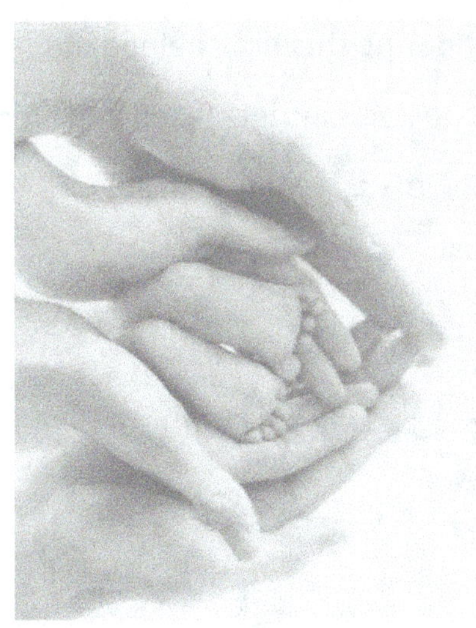

Once the mucus plug is lost, the water from the vagina starts oozing out. It is slightly bloody and comes out in a way that you can't hold it.
You should inform your midwife/doctor once mucus plug or water breaks

My body moved to labour quite quick and within 3 hours of the water breaking and losing the mucus plug, I was in labour. Me and my husband had planned for home birth (we live in a country where this is very common and safe), so when the labour began we informed our midwife (doctor) . She came home and checked me and I was 1cm dilated. You need to be 9-10cm dilated to deliver a baby. It meant I had to wait and bear the labour until I reached the desired dilation. Contractions were happening quite intensely. Contractions feel a bit like period pain but stronger, it feels like someone is pushing the vagina. While the contractions gave a strange feeling, breathing during this time helped me greatly. As time progressed the contractions increased and were 1.5minutes apart along with giving me a feeling to push.

CONTRACTION

Contractions feel like period pain when the blood is coming out of your vagina but this one is 1000 times more painful

The intensity of the contraction keeps increasing and that is how you get more dialeted. When you are 10cm dialeted, a baby can be delivered

They say you are almost in final labour when your contractions are 1 -2 minutes apart. You can use apps like BabyCenter which have the contraction timers to time the contraction.

After bearing the intense contractions for 4.5 hours, we called the midwife again only to find out I was 3 cm dilated. The pain by this point had become unbearable, I was crying. I took a hot shower to ease the pain, kept a hot water bag at various places but nothing seemed to help. With each contraction the pain just seemed to increase but the dilation was not increasing. With the pain getting beyond my bearing power, we decided to go to the hospital. There I was put on monitoring for half an hour to check the baby and my health.

After 30 mins, they said they could give an epidural, which helps reduce the contraction pain. Please know that epidural doesn't work for everybody. Now though I had a go ahead to get an epidural but the doctor who could administer it was not available immediately. It was already 4:30 AM and I was bearing this pain from almost 6 PM. My body was tired and I couldn't take it anymore so I told them to give me anything available. They suggested starting with Morphine and then switching to epidural once the doctor is available. My husband was not convinced but I couldn't bear the pain so we started with morphine. I can't tell you what a relief it was, it instantly helped me and I was better but it made me drowsy. Morphine is known to make you drowsy. The doctor kept me awake full-time. Morphine affects your heart rate and can be dangerous for the baby too. So, when they administer morphine, they ask you not to sleep. It is so difficult to not doze off, but it is critical to be awake.

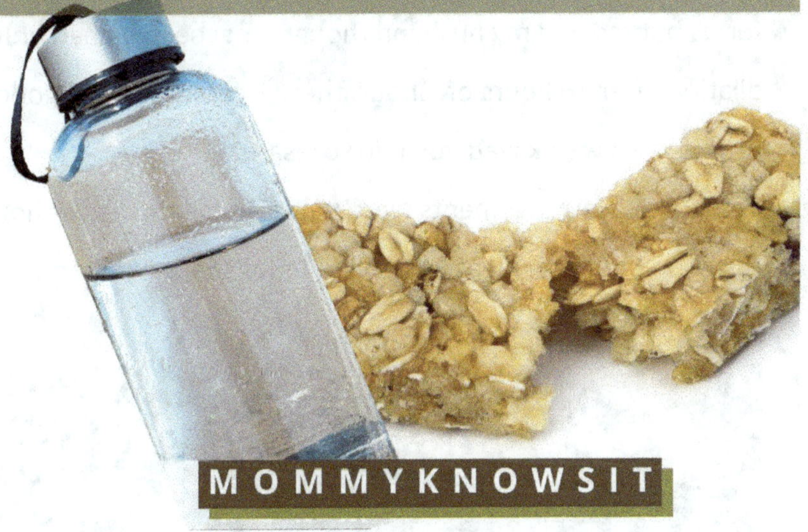

After about an hour the epidural doctor arrived, I was removed from morphine and was put on epidural. Thankfully that helped too and I was in lesser pain. They then asked me to sleep for some time so that my system calms down and hoping the dilation will increase.

I slept for about 2 hours and at 10 AM the doctor checked me, I was 4cm dilated now.

The doctors then told us that they have little hope for normal delivery given the progress with the last 14-16 hours of labour and suggested we opt for Caesarean.

We had not thought about caesarean at all, so it was a tough call for us but me and my husband thought maybe if we had only 4cm dilation after 16 hours of labour, there is less chance of good progress, so we okayed going for caesarean.

Immediately arrangements were made and in the next 2 hours, this little bomb that was troubling me for the last 9 months was out.

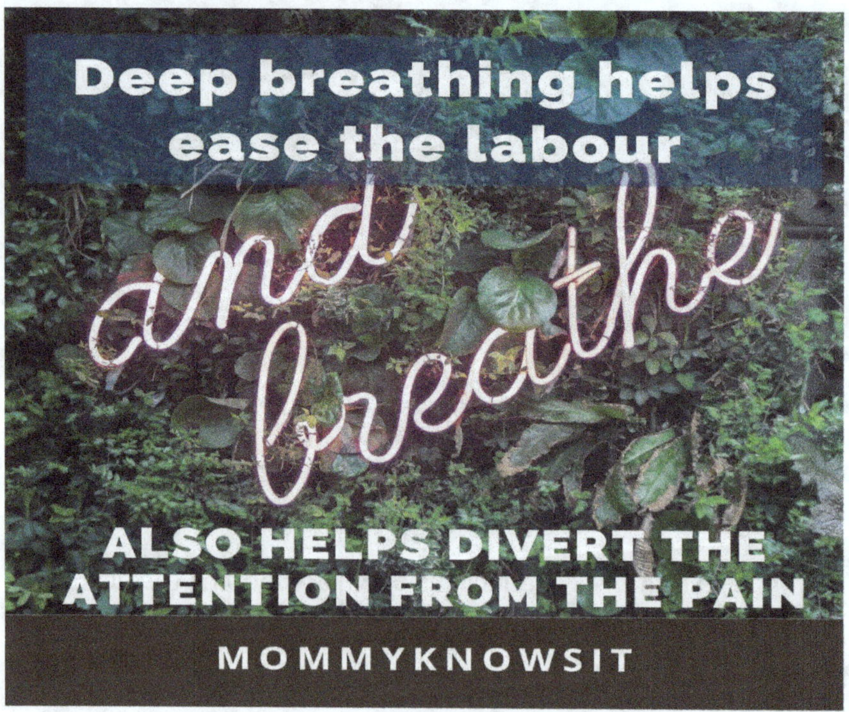

When the doctors got him out and saw he was over 4kgs, they said even if I would have waited for 10 more days, normal delivery would not have gotten him out. I am petite (height wise) so it seems the pelvis would have difficulty to expand so much and it can be tricky (not impossible).

As I was progressing through the pregnancy, each phase had its own challenges but the third trimester felt the toughest. But once I was in labour, the pain was so intense that no day in pregnancy compares to it. The feeling of growing a tiny human inside you is amazIng but labour pain is terrible. So, while I would love to be pregnant 100 times, I would want to skip the labour pain ☺.

Once the baby is out, they give skin to skin with the mom. As it was a c section, they took the baby, cleaned him and then gave skin to skin with his dad until I arrived. I was kept under observation for half an hour and then sent to my hospital room where I had to stay 2 nights. In India, the hospital stay is longer but I stay in the Netherlands where it is 2 nights stay if you undergo a C-Section delivery. The first night, they gave me heavy painkillers and I was not allowed to go to the toilet, they had the arrangement done. The next day everything was removed and the nurse helped me walk, go to the toilet, etc. The hospital tries to get you ready and moving before discharging you. They also provide important guidance on managing the baby and answer queries if you have any.

5: First Month with The Little One

Once your bundle of joy is here, life takes a complete 360-degree shift. Life revolves only around this little wonder that you have just given birth to. They are tiny, they are cute, you want to hold them, cuddle them. It is a beautiful phase but also equally challenging especially for first time parents.

The first three months can be quite tricky with managing the baby, your house, your work especially for first time parents as everything is new. But after the initial months, you get a hang of things and then it is not as terrible as it was in the initial days. In the first few months, the baby sleeps for most of the time so you will have time to do a lot of your work but as they grow their sleep time decreases (during the day) and so you will have less time to do your work. My baby from day 1 said no to sleeping in his crib. I call myself a clingy mom, against my husband's will I said I will co-sleep with my baby. And I don't know about others but it has been one of the best decisions. I love holding my little one, his cuddles, the soft hugs and the smile I get when he wakes up in my arms. I love it but you have to be mindful that this co-sleeping practice takes away a lot of your time so you will have less/no time for your own. Also, you and your husband don't get intimate time due to the presence of the baby in the bed – so co-sleep only if you are ok with it, otherwise put the baby in the habit of sleeping in the crib from the beginning.

> # Trust your instincts as a parent to decide what is right for your baby and what is not!
>
> **MommyKnowsIt**

Post-delivery depression is
real, so if you experience
any sad feeling - don't beat
yourself up!
Talk to your partner, friend,
someone close to you.
Sharing your feelings
during this time help
greatly to keep away from
slipping into depression

Certain things to know as a new mom/dad;

- Babies get rashes (redness) due to the diaper. It is ok, just ensure to give the baby a little diaper free time. 5-10 minutes once or twice when you change the diaper is good enough for the first two months

- Breast milk or Formula milk - both provide all the nutrients to the baby so don't worry if you are not getting breastmilk

- Breast milk is produced from the blood of the mother so what you eat doesn't have an immediate impact on the baby. So, don't worry if the baby has gas, it is not because of your last meal. Babies have tiny tummies that really can't digest easily so they tend to have gas irrespective. What can really help is the activities that help keep gas away – more on that later.

- New born have gas and colic issues in the first 3 months and can sometimes go on until 6-8 months. There is only little that we as parents can do - do it and support your baby through this phase. It is extremely tough to see your little baby in pain and uneasy but we can't do much so try to soothe the baby. Do the activities for gas regularly, this can really help to reduce or ease the process of passing gas

- New born grow with sleep, so ensure the baby sleeps enough and plays a little when awake so that they are tired to sleep

- Don't over/under feed your baby - demand feeding is fine or you can follow the schedule the hospital/paediatrician would give

This little wonder comes with a lot of responsibility. In the initial days, you need to feed them and change their diaper every 2-3 hours. Ensure to burp the baby after every feed - you need not get the burp sound but it is important to do all the burping exercises for 10-15 minutes.

Listing down some of the activities that should/can be done to help the baby burp and pass the gas easily, thus preventing gas issues;

- After every feed, take them on your shoulder and pat them. Do this for 5-10 minutes at minimum. The more time you keep them vertical, the better it is for their food to go down
- Use an anti-colic milk bottle. There are bottles in the market which are designed in such a way that least air goes in the baby mouth while drinking milk, thus helping reduce the gas/uneasiness due to gas
- Tummy time is critical not just to help ease the gas problem but also helps in the baby development. It is good to do tummy time 10-15 minutes everyday
- Lightly massaging the baby tummy in circles around the navel. It is said that this helps release gas if any
- Take the baby legs and gently press them over the tummy. A lot of times, the baby releases gas while doing this
- Hold the baby horizontally as shown in the picture below

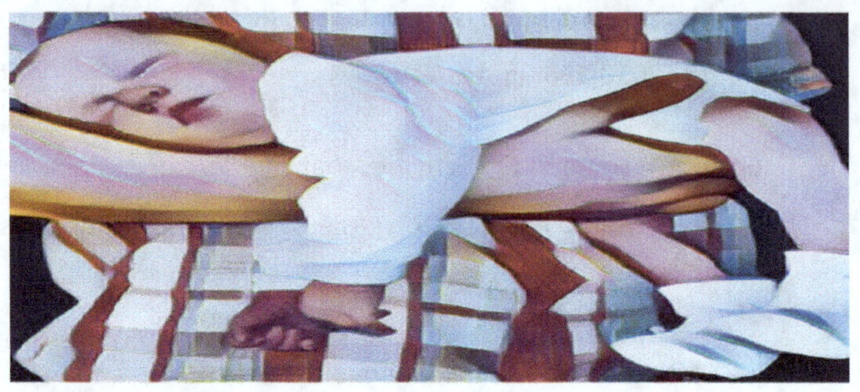

Being abroad where the weather is quite cold, we gave the baby a bath once a week in the initial months - but you can decide the frequency based on what you feel is right for your baby. Frequent bathing should be avoided in the initial days as the baby skin is very tender and can dry out by frequent bathing. In the first 3 months the baby doesn't produce Vitamin K which is needed to heal any internal bleeding that might happen, so give them external Vitamin K supplements (drops).

After delivery, you have a heavy bleeding flow and also the body experiences hormonal changes - now to get itself in the normal stage. So, a lot of women experience depression - people glorify child birth and babies but no one really talks about it. Me and my husband were alone for my baby birth (we live abroad and our families couldn't come), so it was a lot taxing for us to take care of everything. I experienced bouts of depression almost for the first 3-4 months after delivery. Since I had already read a lot about it, the moment I experienced it I acted. I experienced depression from the 4th day after delivery. It used to be a sad feeling that would come for a couple hours and then I would be back to normal. Having known what depression is, I started sharing what I was experiencing with my husband. I also spoke about it with a couple of friends and my doctor. All were very supportive and told me to keep monitoring myself and sharing - as sharing really helps with healing. In normal circumstances if I have any low feeling, I meditate but with a new baby - getting sound sleep was a challenge, meditation would be a far-off dream. Sharing my feelings with close ones, especially my husband, watching my favourite shows, eating my favourite food and loads of cuddles to the little one helped me to crawl through those tough months.

Everyone will have loads of advice for you through pregnancy and once you have the baby but do what you feel is right for the baby. You and your husband/partner have produced the baby and you surely know what works best, so trust your instincts.

As a mother who has gone through hell lot of bodily changes in the last 9 months to make this little human, give yourself and your body time to heal. It takes 9 months to make a baby and 12 - 18 months to heal the body after that. Ensure to give your body and mind that time to heal.

Take the time to heal yourself mentally and physically don't rush the process

It takes 9 months to make a baby and about 18 months to completely heal, give yourself that time!

MOMMYKNOWSIT

6. Take-Away For Each Phase In The Baby Making Journey

Pregnancy, Delivery and Taking Care of the Baby are exceptionally tiring processes and hence taking care of your physical and emotional health are of prime importance.

Here is a list of some Do's and Don'ts that every mother/father should take a note of during each of the periods;

During Pregnancy:

Dos:

- **Attend regular prenatal check-ups:** Schedule and attend all recommended prenatal appointments to monitor the health of both you and your baby.

- **Maintain a balanced diet:** Consume a variety of nutrient-rich foods, including fruits, vegetables, lean proteins, whole grains, and dairy to support your baby's development.

- **Stay hydrated:** Drink plenty of water throughout the day to help with digestion, circulation, and amniotic fluid production.

- **Exercise regularly - But only as much as your body can take or doctor recommended:** Engage in moderate exercise, such as walking, swimming, or prenatal yoga, to promote overall health and reduce the risk of complications.

- **Get enough rest**: Aim for 7-9 hours of quality sleep each night to support your physical and emotional well-being.

- **Take prenatal vitamins:** Ensure you are getting essential nutrients by taking prenatal vitamins as recommended by your healthcare provider.

- **Practice good hygiene:** Wash your hands regularly, especially before eating, to minimize the risk of infections.

- **Educate yourself:** Knowing what to expect during pregnancy, childbirth and postpartum can help ease out a lot of probable stress.

- **Stay positive and manage stress:** Practice relaxation techniques, such as deep breathing and meditation, to manage stress and promote emotional well-being.

- **Communicate with your partner:** Bonding with your partner during and after pregnancy is very important because it is a big change for both of you. Even men go through post-partum depression sometimes so do not discard the connection. Share your feelings, concerns, and expectations with your partner, and work together to create a supportive environment.

- **Wear comfortable clothing and shoes:** As your body changes, opt for comfortable clothing and supportive footwear to reduce discomfort.

- **Practice Kegel exercises:** Strengthen pelvic floor muscles with Kegel exercises to help with bladder control and prepare for natural childbirth.

- **Planning for support:** Having a clear plan of how you plan to take care of the baby helps reduce a lot of hassle in the later phases. Discuss and decide with your partner if you would be getting help from your family or getting a baby-sitter, etc.

Don'ts:

- **Avoid alcohol and tobacco:** Eliminate alcohol and tobacco use during pregnancy to minimize the risk of birth defects and complications.

- **Limit caffeine intake:** Reduce your caffeine intake to a moderate level - you do not need to give it up completely but moderate intake is wise. Excessive caffeine consumption may be associated with an increased risk of miscarriage.

- **Avoid certain foods:** Steer clear of raw or undercooked seafood, unpasteurized dairy products, and other foods that may pose a risk of foodborne illnesses.

- **Say no to high-mercury fish:** Limit the consumption of high-mercury fish like shark, swordfish, king mackerel, and tilefish, as excessive mercury intake can harm the developing nervous system of the baby.

- **Limit exposure to harmful substances**: Minimize exposure to harmful chemicals, such as cleaning products and pesticides, to protect your baby's health.

- **Avoid hot tubs and saunas:** Prolonged exposure to high temperatures can be harmful to the developing fetus, so it's best to avoid hot tubs and saunas.

- **Don't ignore dental care:** Maintain good oral hygiene and attend dental check-ups, as hormonal changes during pregnancy may increase the risk of gum disease.

- **Limit strenuous exercise:** While exercise is important, avoid activities that involve a high risk of falling or injury, and consult your healthcare provider for guidance.

- **Don't skip meals:** Maintain a regular eating schedule to provide your body and baby with consistent nourishment.

- **Avoid excessive weight gain:** While weight gain is expected during pregnancy, excessive gain can lead to complications. Follow your healthcare provider's guidelines.

- **Don't self-diagnose or self-medicate:** Always consult your healthcare provider before taking any medications or supplements, and avoid self-diagnosing medical conditions.

- **Skip risky activities:** Avoid activities that carry a risk of falling or injury, such as contact sports or activities with a high risk of abdominal trauma.

- **Don't delay seeking medical attention**: If you experience unusual symptoms or discomfort, consult your healthcare provider promptly rather than delaying seeking medical attention.

- **Avoid excessive stress:** Chronic stress can have negative effects on pregnancy. Practice stress-management techniques and seek support when needed.

- **Don't ignore signs of preterm labor:** Be aware of the signs of preterm labor, such as regular contractions, abdominal pain, or vaginal bleeding, and seek immediate medical attention if you experience them.

Do's and Don'ts post delivery;

Dos:

- **Rest and recover:** Allow yourself time to rest and recover from the physical and emotional demands of childbirth.

- **Eat a nourishing diet:** Continue to prioritize a balanced diet to support your recovery and provide essential nutrients if you are breastfeeding.

- **Stay hydrated:** Drink plenty of water to support breastfeeding and maintain overall health.

- **Accept help:** Don't hesitate to accept offers of assistance from friends and family. Allow others to help with household chores and daily tasks. Having help for chores is a blessing and will help with your physical recovery.

- **Listen to your body:** Pay attention to your body's signals. Rest when you need to, and don't push yourself too hard.

- **Practice gentle exercises:** Start with gentle postpartum exercises as advised by your healthcare provider to help strengthen your core muscles and improve energy levels.

- **Connect with other moms:** Join local or online support groups to connect with other new moms, share experiences, and gain support. This helps with knowing the common issues babies have, plus having a trusted circle apart from family is good.

- **Prioritize self-care:** Take time for yourself, even if it's just a few minutes each day. This is not taken seriously enough but **ME TIME IS CRITICAL.** Not prioritizing some me time can take a toll on your mental health.

- **Attend postpartum check-ups:** Keep up with postpartum check-ups with your healthcare provider to monitor your physical and emotional well-being.

- **Communicate with your partner:** Maintain open communication with your partner about your needs, feelings, and adjustments as you both adapt to parenthood. Also listen to them since they also go through a lot of emotional upheaval in this entire journey.

- **Establish a routine:** Create a flexible routine that works for you and your baby, including feeding, sleeping, and playtime.

- **Seek professional help if needed:** If you're struggling with postpartum mood disorders or find it challenging to cope, seek professional help from a healthcare provider or counselor. There is no shame in asking for help if needed.

Having depression or mood swings post delivery are very common. Even men go through it. Seeking timely help can save you from long-term mental damage.

- **Bond with your baby:** Spend quality time bonding with your newborn through skin-to-skin contact, cuddling, and talking to them.

- **Plan contraception:** If you're not planning another pregnancy soon, discuss contraception options with your healthcare provider to find a method that suits your needs.

Don'ts:

- **Don't skip meals:** Maintain regular meals to support your energy levels and overall well-being.

- **Avoid excessive physical activity:** While gentle exercise is beneficial, avoid high-intensity workouts until your healthcare provider gives you the green light.

- **Don't ignore signs of postpartum complications:** Be aware of signs of postpartum complications, such *as excessive bleeding, severe pain, or signs of infection. Seek medical attention if you experience* any concerning symptoms.

- **Avoid excessive caffeine and alcohol:** Limit your intake of caffeine and avoid alcohol if you are breastfeeding. If you choose to drink alcohol, do so in moderation.

- **Don't isolate yourself:** Connect with friends and family, and don't isolate yourself. Share your experiences and feelings with your support system.

- **Avoid overcommitting:** Once the baby is out, the new parents get super busy and their schedule becomes unpredictable. Things that were happening in a breeze now take forever, so limit social obligations and commitments during the early weeks postpartum. Focus on rest and bonding with your baby.

- **Don't compare yourself to others:** Every postpartum experience is unique. Avoid comparing yourself to other moms and focus on what works best for you and your baby.

- **Don't neglect your emotional health:** If you're experiencing mood swings, anxiety, or sadness, reach out for emotional support and professional help.

- **Avoid heavy lifting:** Steer clear of heavy lifting during the initial postpartum period, as your body needs time to heal.

- **Don't fuss over breastfeeding:** Having a healthy baby with a full tummy is important, whether it is through breastfeeding or formula feed. Do not stress yourself with breastfeeding. While breastfeeding has a lot of advantages, if you do not get milk, it is absolutely ok. There are a lot of babies who have grown without breastmilk and are healthy and hearty, so your baby is not losing anything. Spend time with the baby, cuddle them, hug them and you will have a happy baby.

- **Avoid tight clothing:** Opt for loose and comfortable clothing to avoid unnecessary pressure on healing areas, especially if you've had a cesarean section.

- **Don't skip postpartum pelvic floor exercises:** Pelvic floor exercises can aid in recovery, especially if you've had a vaginal delivery. Consult with your healthcare provider for guidance.

- **Avoid excessive worrying:** While it's natural to be concerned about your baby, try to manage worry and stress to promote a positive postpartum experience.

- **Avoid delaying contraception discussions:** Discuss contraception options with your healthcare provider in a timely manner to avoid unplanned pregnancies.

Do's and Don'ts with a New-Born;

Dos:

- **Feed on demand**: Whether breastfeeding or formula-feeding, respond to your baby's hunger cues and feed them on demand. Don't force feed the baby.

- **Practice safe sleep:** Always place your baby on their back to sleep and ensure they have a firm mattress with no loose bedding or toys in the crib.

- **Keep the baby warm:** Dress your baby appropriately for the temperature and use lightweight blankets to keep them warm while avoiding overheating.

- **Hold and cuddle your baby:** Newborns thrive on physical contact. Hold, cuddle, and provide skin-to-skin contact to foster a sense of security and bonding.

- **Maintain good hygiene**: Keep your baby clean by bathing them regularly, cleaning their diaper area, and trimming their nails carefully.

- **Follow a sleep routine:** Establish a bedtime routine to help your baby distinguish between day and night. Keep nighttime feedings calm and low-key.

- **Talk and sing to your baby:** Engage in gentle conversation and sing lullabies to stimulate your baby's developing senses and promote language development.

- **Burp your baby:** After feedings, gently burp your baby to help prevent discomfort and reduce the likelihood of spit-up.

- **Create a safe environment:** Baby-proof your home by securing furniture, covering electrical outlets, and keeping small objects out of reach.

- **Follow vaccination schedules:** Keep up with your baby's immunization schedule as recommended by your pediatrician to protect them from preventable diseases.

- **Monitor your baby's development:** Keep track of developmental milestones and discuss any concerns with your pediatrician during regular check-ups.

- **Provide tummy time:** Allow your baby supervised tummy time when they are awake to help strengthen their neck and shoulder muscles.

- **Accept help:** Don't hesitate to accept assistance from friends and family. Taking care of a newborn is a team effort.

- **Trust your instincts:** You know your baby best. Trust your instincts and seek guidance from healthcare professionals when needed.

Don'ts:

- **Don't overbundle:** Avoid overdressing your baby, and be mindful of signs of overheating, such as sweating or feeling hot to the touch.

- **Avoid exposure to sick individuals:** Limit your baby's exposure to sick individuals, especially during the early months when their immune system is still developing.

- **Don't shake your baby:** Never shake your baby. Shaking can cause serious brain injuries. If you're feeling overwhelmed, put the baby down in a safe place and take a moment to collect yourself.

- **Don't put objects in the crib:** Avoid placing soft toys, pillows, or loose bedding in the crib to reduce the risk of Sudden Infant Death Syndrome (SIDS).

- **Don't delay diaper changes:** Change your baby's diaper promptly to prevent diaper rash and discomfort.

- **Avoid smoking around your baby:** Secondhand smoke is harmful to infants and increases the risk of respiratory issues and SIDS.

- **Don't skip tummy time:** Tummy time is crucial for your baby's development. Don't neglect this activity during awake periods.

- **Avoid overstimulation:** Newborns can easily become overstimulated. Provide a calm environment and pay attention to your baby's cues to avoid sensory overload.

- **Don't use unnecessary products:** Limit the use of baby products to essential items. Avoid using strong fragrances or unnecessary chemicals on your baby's delicate skin.

- **Avoid exposure to direct sunlight:** Protect your baby's sensitive skin from direct sunlight. If you need to be outdoors, use baby-safe sunscreen and dress your baby in lightweight, long-sleeved clothing and a hat.

- **Avoid placing your baby on soft surfaces:** Place your baby on a firm mattress for sleep, and avoid placing them on soft surfaces such as sofas or waterbeds.

If you are healthy physically and mentally, you can take great care of your baby and raise a healthy child. So always ensure to take care of yourself along with the baby.

Follow @MommyKnowsIt on Instagram/Facebook for tips & tricks on pregnancy, child birth and post-delivery

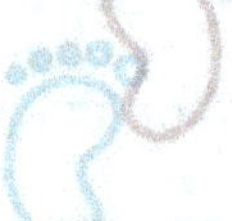

www.ingramcontent.com/pod-product-compliance
Lightning Source LLC
Chambersburg PA
CBHW050735260726